THE AMERICAN MEDICAL ASSOCIATION AND ORGANIZED MEDICINE

ORGANIZATIONS AND INTEREST GROUPS
(VOL. 8)

GARLAND REFERENCE LIBRARY
OF SOCIAL SCIENCE
(VOL. 713)

Organizations and Interest Groups
Series Editor: James S. Bowman

The General Accounting Office:
An Annotated Bibliography
Robert L. Hollings

The American Civil Liberties Union:
An Annotated Bibliography
Samuel Walker

Public Interest Law: An Annotated Bibliography and Research Guide
Lee Epstein, Tracey E. George, and Joseph F. Kobylka

Interest Groups: An Annotated Bibliography
Allan J. Cigler, Raymond Birt, and Anthony J. Nownes

Nonprofit Public Policy Research Organizations:
A Sourcebook on Think Tanks in Government
Robert L. Hollings

The American Medical Association and
Organized Medicine: A Commentary
and Annotated Bibliography
James A. Johnson, Walter J. Jones

THE AMERICAN MEDICAL ASSOCIATION AND ORGANIZED MEDICINE

A Commentary and Annotated Bibliography

James A. Johnson

Walter J. Jones

GARLAND PUBLISHING, INC. • NEW YORK & LONDON
1993

Library of Congress Cataloging-in-Publication Data

Johnson, James A., 1954–
The American Medical Association and organized medicine : a commentary and annotated bibliography / by James A. Johnson, Walter J. Jones.
p. cm. — (Garland reference library of social science : vol. 713) (Organizations and interest groups : vol. 8)
Includes index.
ISBN 0–8153–0049–2 (alk. paper)
1. American Medical Association. 2. American Medical Association—Bibliography. I. Jones, Walter J. II. Title. III. Series. IV. Series: Garland reference library of social science : v. 713.
[DNLM: 1. American Medical Association. 2. Societies, Medical—history—United States. 3. Societies, Medical—United States—abstracts. WB 1 AA1 A5J 1993]
R15.J64 1993
610'.6'073—dc20
DNLM/DLC
for Library of Congress 93–7145
CIP

Printed on acid-free, 250-year-life paper
Manufactured in the United States of America

Series Foreword

The modern era is one of organizations, and as we approach the next century there is little evidence that the importance of institutions in society will diminish. As they have grown in scope and number so has material published by and about them. Yet managers, academicians and their students, and researchers do not have ready access to information about these significant social entities. In an increasingly complex world of organizations, more and more people need such data to assist in defining and solving problems.

The lack of a comprehensive information system has frustrated users, disseminators, and generators of knowledge; the documentation and control of the literature on organizations have been generally neglected. Indeed, major gaps in the development of the literature, the bibliographical structure of the field, have evolved.

Garland Publishing, Inc., has inaugurated the present series as an authoritative guide to information sources on the subject. It seeks to consolidate published material on a wide variety of public, private, and nonprofit organizations including: (a) federal agencies, congressional committees, the judicial branch, and international bodies; (b) corporations, interest groups, trade unions, and consulting firms; as well as (c) professional associations, scientific societies, and educational institutions.

Each book will be compiled by one or more specialists in the area. The authors—practitioners and scholars—are selected in open competition from across the country. They design their work to include an introductory essay, a wide variety of bibliographic materials, and, where appropriate, an information resource section. Thus each contribution in the collection provides a systematic basis for managers and researchers to make informed judgments in the course of their work.

Since no single volume can adequately encompass such a broad, interdisciplinary subject, the series is intended as a continuous project that will incorporate new bodies of literature as needed. Its titles represent the initial building blocks in an operating information system for understanding organizations and society. As an open-ended endeavor, it is hoped that not only will the series serve to summarize knowledge in the field but also will contribute to its advancement.

This collection of book-length bibliographies is the product of considerable collaboration on the part of many people. Special appreciation is extended to the individual contributors in the series and to the anonymous reviewers of each of the volumes. Inquiries should be made to the Series Editor.

James S. Bowman
School of Public Administration and Policy
Florida State University

Contents

Acknowledgments

Many people contributed to the accomplishment of this very challenging task. We want to thank James Bowman, Ph.D., at Florida State University for being a supportive editor who was there when we needed him but left us alone otherwise. Thanks to Michael Samuels, Dr.P.H. at the University of South Carolina for his insightful review and suggestions. We are most grateful to Lester King, M.D., a renowned medical historian who was so gracious with his time and knowledge. The library staff at the AMA and at the Medical University of South Carolina deserve our thanks for their many hours of assistance. However, the most invaluable people of all were our many research assistants.

We had a curious sequence of events that led to constant churning of our research staff. Our first research assistant was Dan Gentry who was accepted into the Ph.D. program at Berkeley and left for the west coast; the next two were John Schultz and David Manzi, both of whom were called out to Desert Storm. Then came Bill Helfenstein, who was most helpful in organizing what seemed to be a very disorganized project. We lost him when a corporation offered him a position paying about a million times more than we could. After Bill was George Jarriel, who worked like a real trooper until he fell in our office parking lot and fractured his leg in several places. Between the pain medications and his difficulty in getting around, George had to bow out.

In the final stage, an angel came to our rescue in the form of Sally Miller. Under her leadership and tireless commitment to the project we were able to meet deadlines and assure the quality needed in such an undertaking. Lastly, we would like to thank Duffy Newman for her assistance in carrying the project over the finish line.

Preface

"History offers the best training for those who would take part in public affairs." -Polybius: Historics I, c. 125 BC

The United States is beginning a period with the potential for major change in its health care delivery system. Forces set loose in the 1960s with the introduction of Medicare and Medicaid have combined to produce a system that leaves 38 million people with no health insurance, another major group underinsured, and soaring insurance costs for those with "adequate" insurance. There is a clear need for reform of the health care system. It is important, not only to have good analysis of the current health care delivery system, but to understand how it got that way. The only way to understand the current situation is to understand its history. The history must also be understood in the context of the times in which it evolved and the broader social, economic, and political trends that define us as a people. Only then is it possible to frame reforms that will meet the health care needs of the American people and be accepted by the public, the health professionals, and related special interests. To support historically derived public policy it is critical that the analyst have access to historical materials presented in a manner that facilitates good scholarship. You will find that this book does exactly that by providing the critical readings for each era after setting the social, political, and economic context for the reader. Also provided is an overview introduction that places the total work in context and a concluding chapter with speculation about the future of "organized medicine" in the U.S. health care system.

The book is especially relevant to health care reform in the United States because it focuses on the major catalyst of the U.S. health care system. This unique catalyst is the American Medical Association ("organized medicine"). The book and its readings show how the American Medical Association (AMA) evolved and shaped our current system. The system they helped to create is the only one in the world with such a heavy reliance on private practitioners, historically late evolution of health insurance and lack of universal coverage , and private sector dominance of the health services delivery system. This evolution has made American physicians relatively more prestigious and economically advantaged than their counterparts anywhere else in the world, but the US lags behind many countries in outcomes like average length of life and infant death rates. The book provides insights into how that came to be.

The book and its readings will be of primary interest to professors and students in the health sciences at the graduate and undergraduate levels as a text book and or resources book for teaching health care history, policy and politics. It will also be of interest to professors and students of public policy and history.

The availability of this information in the format presented here opens the door for the application of historical interpretation of the evolution of the U.S. health care system to current public policy debates. I hope it will be a catalyst and major resource for health policy analysts, both academic and applied, dedicated to the development of good public policy for the reform of the American health care system. Formulating good public policy in health care is only possible if we know: who we are as people, the evolution of the current health care system and the forces that shaped it, and the forces surrounding the current system. I believe that this book and is the first small step in facilitating the scholarship and interest to promote a truly informed public debate on health care reform.

Michael E. Samuels, Dr. P.H.

Part One

Historical Background of the AMA and Organized Medicine

1

INTRODUCTION AND CHRONOLOGY

Health Care, American Society and the AMA

Observers of America as varied as Alexis DeTocqueville, Karl Marx and David Truman have noted the prevalence and importance of organized interest groups in every sector of society. U.S. political and economic activities are largely dominated by interest groups, and most citizens are formal or de facto members (however attenuated) of one or more associations of like-minded and/or like-interested members. Conflicts among interest groups, and the rise and fall of dominant groups and coalitions of groups, illustrate the basic historical and social evolution of the nation.

The health care sector in the United States is no less politicized than other parts of American society, though citizens have sometimes tried to think of health care as "above politics" (just as, until the rise of persistent cost inflation, they have often wished it to be "above economics"). U.S. health care, however, is exceptional in one significant way. Few other components of modern America can be so clearly tied to the efforts and fortunes of one particular interest group--the American Medical Association (AMA). Indeed, as the totality of the readings covered in this book demonstrates, the successful politics practiced by the AMA is primarily responsible for most of the features of American health care that set it off from corresponding systems in such countries as Canada and the United Kingdom. These include the heavy reliance on fee-for-service physicians, the historically recent development of health insurance programs (as compared to other industrialized nations) and private sector dominance of the service delivery system (though not, increasingly, the payment system).

When Americans talk of "organized medicine", they are generally thinking of the AMA. Their vision is of wealthy and influential doctors, pillars of the established order of things. Why and how have

U.S. physicians, working through the AMA, been so successful in establishing and maintaining an elite position of economic prosperity and political power? The readings covered in this book demonstrate that there is no one explanation for this outcome.

As health services scholars who have examined the history and functioning of the AMA in great detail, we would argue that the rise to power of the AMA can be best thought of as a result of a complex interaction of professional ambition, organizational development, and national evolution. The American Medical Association was historically able to develop and maintain organizational cohesion (Burrow, 1963) and (more importantly) professional consensus on desirable public and occupational policies (Feldstein, 1977). At times, the organization has been blessed with very skillful leadership (Campion, 1984). The growth of a technologically dynamic and sophisticated health care sector — along with a large and rich nation which could pay the resulting bills — also enabled American doctors to gain power. The AMA has also benefited from (and actively worked at sustaining) a generally positive public attitude toward the physician profession (Capuzzi, 1980).

Yet we note that most other socioeconomically advanced nations have possessed many of the same conditions, but none have such an influential physicians' organization. Part of the answer to the question of AMA power undoubtedly stems from unique national social, political and economic factors. After all, the United States has always been unique in its support of the ideologies of private enterprise and individualism, and so reveres physician autonomy, and the one-on-one physician-patient relationship.

As a nation born in rebellion against perceived imperial tyranny, the United States has also been suspicious of governmental intervention into the actual workings of the health care sector. Thus, until the 1940's, kept the most obvious national counterweight to physician power — the federal government — out of the medical arena. Doctors, and the AMA, therefore had a largely free hand in establishing a health care system with themselves at its pinnacle. In contrast, English physicians (and the British Medical Association), existing within a more communally-oriented society, had to accept the establishment of the National Health Service after the Second World War.

Some of the AMA's distinctiveness comes as well from its own efforts. The Association has a popular image of status quo rigidity. Yet, like all other interest groups that have been successful in dominating their corner of society, the AMA has a history of growth and change. As Fishbein (1947) and Holler (1981) describe, the Association's humble origins (born in a log cabin, figuratively speaking) belie its widely-perceived elite status.

Social, economic and technological changes in the U.S. health care system are transforming the nature of American health care, and the AMA, as they did at the beginning of the century. Indeed, neither the AMA's strongest supporters, or its most strident critics (each side being well represented in this book) seem to fully appreciate how much the position of the AMA has changed from the era of its unopposed dominance. To maintain its viability, the Association has altered itself and its policy positions markedly in recent years. (For example, it has moved from diehard opposition to national health insurance to advocacy of its own NHI proposal.) Given continuing pressures, this organizational evolution will undoubtedly have to continue (James, 1988; AMA, 1987). AMA advocates must recognize that its era of health systems dominance has ended forever. But the Association's opponents should not underestimate its demonstrated survival instincts — its ability to change, however belatedly, to meet new times and new challenges (Ginzberg, 1977).

In fact, the growth and evolution of the AMA over the last century and a half provide us with a superb illustration of the potentialities and limitations of interest group power within a modern democratic society. The history of the AMA shows us that groups that organize social institutions to create change and gain power are themselves integrally transformed by the process. The act of control sets chains of events in motion that lead to unanticipated as well as expected results. From then on, the dominance of any organization, however powerful, is challenged by patterns of social evolution that it cannot completely control. As pluralist political theory would suggest, the only constant is change--with political power as with everything else.

The Origins and Development of the AMA

The American Medical Association was founded in 1847, when most American medicine was considered second-rate even by nineteenth - century standards. As authors such as Kaufman (1976), Kett (1968), and Shafer (1968) point out, American doctors had no standardized training, and each state had its own requirements (often virtually non-existent) for licensure. When combined with primitive science and technology, their efforts were often more damaging to the patient than the original malady for which the patient was being treated. Most physicians had low incomes, and wealthier and more educated citizens preferred treatment by European doctors (ideally, in Europe).

The founders of the AMA wanted things to be different. They wanted physicians to be well-paid, well-educated and respected members of the community (Shryock, 1960). They were alarmed that there was little national consensus over what a trained physician should be. American medicine was highly diversified, with "sects" and "schools" of all description, preaching and practicing a wide range of ideologies, spiritualisms, and physical principles. The AMA wanted a unified physician profession that would gain respect for effective treatment based upon the most up-to-date scientific principles. In their belief in science, these physician reformers were solidly behind a "progressive" movement that included evolutionists, industrial management advocates, modern educators, and public health crusaders.

Progressivism would significantly change the face of America in the first years of the twentieth century. Until its triumph, however, the AMA weathered a difficult fifty years. It worked with other like-minded organizations in state after state to tighten licensure standards, and energetically promoted higher and more uniform standards of medical education (Duffy, 1976). Progress was slow but steady. By 1900, the progressive movement had advanced on all fronts. As President, Theodore Roosevelt would strongly push for the kinds of health regulations (exemplified by the Pure Food and Drug Act) that the AMA advocated. American society in general was enamoured of scientific and technological development and organization, equating them with national power and prosperity.

With this social climate, the AMA, and its Council on Medical Education, made more rapid process in molding medical education and practice to its own liking. To be sure, almost all of the significant reforms and innovations in medical school curriculum and management came from outside of the AMA (Ludmerer, 1985). Nevertheless, the AMA was able to identify its cause with these reforms, and use them to advance its own agenda of professional primacy within health care. Like other ambitious interest groups, the Association had found that the selective development and use of alliances with other social forces was essential to gaining power.

The culmination of the reform efforts came between 1910 and 1920. The famous report on American medical education by Abraham Flexner in fact provided little truly new information about the state of medical education (Berliner, 1977). The uneven and often low standards seen in medical schools had been observed and deplored by many medical professionals and educators for some time (Hunt, 1991). However, the Flexner Report was a classic case of research gaining influence through release at the right time, into the right hands. In the final decade of progressivism, the states responded to the report's scandalous findings with a wave of regulation that implemented the unified medical education model that the AMA and others advocated (Burrow, 1977). Unorthodox practices were proscribed; the educational variations represented by the proprietary medical schools were ended - along with most of the proprietary schools.

By 1920, a monolithic structure of "scientific medical education" was largely in place. Physicians were at the pinnacle of the structure (Starr, 1982). And the chief interest group organization for these physicians was the AMA. The AMA had attained its goal of professional domination not through sheer force of numbers, or even explicit approval from a national majority of citizens or their representatives. Instead, the Association had joined a larger progressive coalition, and facilitated its movement toward ends that would benefit the AMA more than the other coalition members.

AMA power extended to all parts of health care, not simply those aspects that directly concerned physicians. Between 1920 and 1960, the Association gained official representative status on a wide range of state and federal government boards and regulatory agencies. The Joint Commission on Accreditation of Health Organizations (JCAHO), which monitors the operating standards of health facilities and has the power to financially cripple any wayward organization through a negative report, has AMA members in its central governing body. Most educational accrediting agencies have AMA members on their governing boards, even those that have authority over the training of other health professionals such as allied health practitioners (Weithaus and Fauser, 1991). Quite literally, the AMA and its members were given a nearly free hand to shape all significant aspects of U.S. health care for two generations.

Growing Challenges to AMA Power

Despite their avowed reluctance to engage in the grubbiness of politics (as opposed to the sanctified practice of "scientific" patient care), the leaders of the AMA had turned out to be some of the most successful interest group politicians in American history (Hyde et al., 1984; Keiser and Jones, 1986; Kronenfeld and Whicker, 1984). Ironically, given the stark ideological differences, the AMA's use of a wider coalition to gain power for itself was political activism as skillful as that employed by the Leninists to capture control of Russia during the same time period. And in a similar (though certainly more benign and socially beneficial) way, it resulted in near-total control.

As suggested earlier, however, the most successful interest groups find that their very success creates new and often more difficult challenges than those found while still in opposition to the established order. Put another way, the tasks of maintaining power are quite different from those of gaining power (Campion, 1984). Even during the period of consolidation that lasted from the 1920s until World War II, the power of physicians and the AMA was increasingly questioned. Progressivism as a political and social movement had largely dissipated by the Twenties, and the progressive image (and, to a significant extent, behavior) of the AMA faded as well. The organization had been victorious in creating a new status quo in health care, and was now identified as a chief component of the medical establishment. It could be blamed (rightly or wrongly) for a wide variety of social ills, and the undeniable deficiencies of American health care. The enormous prosperity of physicians seemed unjust to many in a society with millions of medically indigent citizens.

The power of the AMA was also gradually weakened by an increasingly inhospitable social and technological environment. The "scientific medicine" promoted by progressivism led to technological innovation and development that inevitably required larger amounts of capital, and industrial concentration (Lewis and Steps, 1983). As with other economic sectors, advances turned health care into "big business", whether or not its chief practitioners were willing to admit it (Starr, 1982). The domination of the AMA by private-sector, fee-for-service, solo practicing physicians led to a neglect and denigration of the doctors working in the fast growing sectors of public health, group and salaried practice, and university research (Fox, 1986). Most importantly, the AMA hierarchy was seen as increasingly unsympathetic and irrelevant by the physician specialists that evolved directly from the advances of "scientific medicine". By permitting membership attrition and fragmentation, the AMA committed a mortal sin that no dominant interest group could afford in the long run (Feldstein, 1988).

The stability of the status quo in American society and health care that characterized the 1920s–a status quo that the AMA was partly responsible for and benefited from–was further undermined by the challenges of economic depression and world war in the next twenty-five years. The Great Depression had created a new national consensus for change, and newly-elected President Franklin Roosevelt responded (as had his relative Theodore during his term of office) with a burst of liberal domestic policy making.

Preoccupied with the daunting task of bringing about national economic recovery, FDR took pains not to directly confront the AMA, consulting its leadership before proposing major social legislation such as the Social Security Act of 1935 (Poen, 1979). But the ascendance of the Democratic Party and the New Deal had also brought a large number of more liberal Congressmen and administrators to Washington along with Roosevelt. To the horror of the AMA, they were soon energetically advancing proposals for increased governmental involvement within health care, most prominently through the administration of a system of national health insurance. The general assumption that government had a basic responsibility to ensure that all citizens had at least minimally adequate access to health care became part of the national consensus. (Of course, this did not prevent ongoing and vigorous disagreement about exactly how or to what extent government should fulfill its responsibility.)

During the Thirties, the AMA was able to skillfully construct and hold together interest group coalitions that were able to beat back the liberal proposals (Weeks and Berman, 1985). Led by determined leaders like Morris Fishbein, the AMA held onto its power, and survived challenges such as a celebrated antitrust suit brought against it by the federal government (Fishbein, 1947). Presidential activism might have tipped the political balance against the AMA, but the growing storm clouds of war developing over Europe and Asia turned FDR's attention away from domestic affairs for the rest of his administration (Poen, 1979).

On the surface, U.S. entry into World War II in 1941 took national health care reform from the top of the public agenda. But in fact the massive American mobilization transformed all sectors of society, including health care. Between 1941 and 1945, the United States became the greatest economic and military superpower in history. The federal government became integrally involved in most significant productive activities. The military medical system became the largest health care entity in U.S. history, and thousands of postwar health administrators got their practical training managing huge military medical complexes.

World War II placed the federal government permanently into national health care management. This status was ratified by such postwar legislation as the Hill-Burton Act, which, for the first time, centrally involved the federal government in both public and private sector health facilities development (Stevens, 1989). The growing public appetite for modern health care — an appetite stimulated by the AMA, among others — required health services that could not be provided without large public subsidies (Fox, 1986; Rothstein, 1987). And, as any student of government will point out, sooner or later, issues of subsidy bring on questions of control.

The American Medical Association had succeeded in establishing primacy in health care, but the continual modernization that it supported inevitably brought new and powerful actors into the policy arena. With its solo-practitioner dominated leadership, the organization was faced with the rise of an increasingly bureaucratized and centralized health care sector. How could such a technologically sophisticated and organizationally complex area of society continue to be run with generalist physicians holding such a preponderance of power at the top? As had occurred (and continues to occur; think of the case of Soviet Communism mentioned earlier) with many other entrenched political elites in history, the social structures that the AMA controlled had evolved beyond its ability to control them. New elites were developing in areas such as insurance, facilities planning and management, and technology development and application. Like the AMA before them, they wanted power within the health care sector.

As Burrow (1963) and Campion (1984) note, a number of AMA leaders saw the trends developing and warned their physician members of the threats to their professional prerogatives and hegemony. Faced with slipping membership and increasingly serious financial problems, however, the Association failed to grasp the larger issues at stake. In 1948, it threw its resources into supporting Republican candidates for Congress and the White House, but Roosevelt's Democratic successor, Harry S Truman, was reelected with a Democratic Congress. The AMA was successful in preventing the adoption of Truman's national health insurance proposals, mounting an effective public relations campaign (Poen, 1979). However, this did not stop the more basic changes occurring in the nation's health care system.

In the 1950s, major health reform efforts diminished with the arrival of Republican President Dwight Eisenhower (who received strong AMA support). Eisenhower opposed any significant intrusion of the federal government into the area of health insurance, and gave vocal support to private sector health care. The physician profession itself was still held in high esteem by the public. Physicians as individual professionals became wealthier, even if the AMA as an organization did not. On the surface, the Fifties appeared to be another Republican-led "return to normalcy". But, the decade also brought continued expansion of federal aid programs - again, generally supported by the AMA.

Many of these programs aimed at expanding the production of health professionals to staff the increased supply of hospitals resulting from the Hill-Burton Act. In the 1910 - 1920 period, the AMA had successfully worked to limit the number of physicians through the Flexner-inspired reduction in the nation's medical schools (Burrow, 1977). However, after decades of opposing more medical schools, and larger graduating classes of physicians, the AMA reversed itself and cautiously accepted arguments that the U.S. needed more physicians (Lewis, Fein and Mechanic, 1976). More and more of these new physicians became specialists who declined to affiliate with the AMA, thus accelerating the downward trend in membership. At the end of the Fifties, doctors had more prestige and higher incomes than ever before. But the AMA still had not faced the central political issues that resulted from increasing challenges to physician authority within the health care sector (Burrow, 1963).

The Sixties were a watershed decade for both the U.S. health care system and the American Medical Association. John Kennedy, an activist Democrat, was elected President in 1960. Like Truman (the last Democratic occupant of the White House), he energetically campaigned for increased federal involvement in health care. His primary proposal was not a general national health insurance program, but one targeting the elderly. The distinction was politically crucial. A program for only one social group would inevitably have lower cost estimates, thus blunting charges of fiscal impracticality. In addition, a focus on one identifiable group of beneficiaries is almost always more likely to receive effective political support than one spread out over the entire public. In this case, it was also helpful that the elderly tend to follow public affairs more closely, and vote more consistently, than any other social group.

As in the past, the AMA launched a nationwide campaign against the Medicare proposal. But this time, the Association's leadership realized how their organization's political position had relatively deteriorated since the conflicts of the late Forties. Consequently, the AMA felt obliged, for the first time, to offer a significant counterproposal to Kennedy's program — the "medicredit" plan (Strickland, 1972; Marmor and Christianson, 1982).

This major change in tactics was a sign of potential strength as well as actual weakness. As suggested earlier, the AMA had generally been politically inflexible and reactionary toward reform ideas since gaining health care preeminence in the Twenties. But the organization now finally realized the need to adapt to altered circumstances. New leadership saw that judicious acceptance of change, and compromise with reform advocates, might in fact enhance the AMA's ability to retain effective control over the ultimate course of change (Campion, 1984). What in the past could be done directly, with brute political force, now had to be done indirectly, with a sophisticated strategy of support for conservatively-inclined reform.

The new philosophy of the AMA leadership yielded no immediate political rewards. Efforts to promote "medicredit" went for naught, and President Kennedy did not have the political ability to force his own proposals through Congress (Harris, 1966). As often happens in politics, the stalemate was finally broken not by conscious political strategy on either side, but events outside of the policy arena — in this case, the assassination of President Kennedy in 1963.

In Lyndon Johnson, the AMA faced a far more skillful political operator. The new Chief Executive possessed a legendary ability to twist congressional arms to get what he wanted. In addition, a wave of sympathy and patriotic "rally round the flag" support made Johnson politically invulnerable in the next presidential election. In 1964, President Johnson won in an enormous landslide. His coattails brought dozens of new liberal Democrats into Congress, and decimated the ranks of conservative Republicans. The congressional impasse was broken, and 1965 became a year of dramatic legislative activism. Not only was Medicare adopted, but a new federal and state government initiative to provide health care for the poor was passed - Medicaid (Weeks and Berman, 1985).

Yet, with its ranks of political supporters thinner than ever before, the AMA's strategy of cooptation through cooperation finally began to bear fruit. AMA representatives actively negotiated with the Johnson Administration and congressional members over the details of Medicare and Medicaid, and were able to preserve the central elements of physician dominance in health services delivery - the fee-for-service system, and freedom of physician selection for the patient, in particular (Ginzberg, 1977). In fact, with their acceptance of prevailing and "reasonable" fee scales, the new programs actually placed a taxpayer-funded floor under the income of participating physicians (Califano, 1986).

Medicare and Medicaid did in fact subsidize critically-needed health care for the poor and elderly. But they also evolved with minimal governmental controls over how their funds were in fact spent. For the first time, doctors were able to gain patients and income (in some cases, become millionaires) through the adroit tapping of the federal treasury. Physicians as directly benefited from federal and state spending as did the intended program recipients. If this was how national health reform was to be handled in the United States, it was clear that physicians and the AMA could live with it — indeed, thrive with it (Marmor, 1983).

The Growing Cost Containment Crisis and the AMA

For the next fifteen years (1965 - 1980), physicians did well professionally and economically. New technologies continued to rapidly extend medical capabilities. With its new leadership, the AMA itself began to recover financially, and membership losses were slowed if not eliminated. As it had before, the Association was again instrumental in defeating efforts in the early Seventies to enact a national health insurance program (most prominently, the Kennedy-Corman proposal).

If there was any flaw in the AMA conservative reform strategy that had brought about such results, it was its very success. The health care sector, still dominated by physicians, began to extract resources from the rest of the economy at accelerating rates. This rapid increase in health care spending ignited a cost inflation that is still with us. This in turn has brought about cost containment imparatives that now constitute the greatest threat to physician autonomy and AMA power.

The seventies saw continual and severe cost overruns for both Medicare and Medicaid. The increased access to health care that both represent placed upward pressures on costs that strained governmental resources. By the mid-Seventies, federal and state policymakers were actively considering possible means of containing costs (Starr, 1982). As with the enaction of Medicare and Medicaid, the AMA did not (and could not) openly oppose the general concept. In a coalition that included other health industry groups such as the American Hospital Association, it could nevertheless insist that any cost controls preserve private sector health care, the fee-for-service practice, and traditional physician-patient autonomy in establishing relationships (Nesbitt, 1978).

To outside observers, and federal policymakers, it appeared to effectively preclude any truly successful cost containment. The heart of the problem was that U.S. health care had become generally insulated from conventional economic forces by the mid-seventies (Feldstein, 1977). The widespread use of third-party insurance had eliminated normal consumer resistance to price increases. At the political level, Medicare had become a sacrosanct "entitlement" for its primarily white, elderly (and regularly voting) middle-class recipients. All of this might not have mattered in principle; after all, health care has always been treated somewhat specially in modern societies. But in practice, given the modern high technology orientation of American medicine, the removal of marketplace constraints was financially disastrous.

From a political standpoint, the costs imposed on other social actors - corporations that paid the insurance premiums for their employees, in particular - led hitherto-uninvolved groups into the health policy arena. By the late Seventies, the AMA and other health industry groups were facing more powerful political opponents than ever before. Government, business, taxpayers, even patients (who were subjected to increasingly large deductibles and copayments by their insurers) swelled the cost containment constituency.

The Nixon and Ford Administrations had attempted various schemes to control inflation (including, in the case of Nixon, general wage and price controls that included health care), but none had any lasting impact. President Jimmy Carter and his activist Secretary of Health, Education and Welfare, Joseph Califano, proposed more direct controls on hospital charges (Califano 1986). In alliance with the AHA, the American Medical Association defeated the Carter Administration initiatives in Congress. But the medical industry alternative - voluntary price restraints - was completely ineffective. By 1980, health care costs were clearly out of control.

Along with much of the rest of the American public, the AMA and its membership were dissatisfied with the Carter Administration's performance, and undoubtedly a majority of AMA members voted for his conservative Republican opponent, former California Governor Ronald Reagan in 1980. The general assumption was that a pro-business Republican president would be less inclined to propose restrictions on the behavior of health care providers, especially doctors

(Kelly, 1981). The incoming president had repeatedly extolled the virtues of free enterprise, and had declared government to be the problem rather than the solution.

Once in office, however, the Reagan Administration had to also concern itself with the overall budgetary situation for the federal government. It was alarming, as David Stockman, Director of the Office of Management and Budget, later admitted. President Reagan had committed himself to a massive defense buildup, an equally dramatic cut in federal income tax rates, and protection of the "social safety net" (which in practice meant the middle class "entitlements", including Medicare). This path led to large and growing federal budget deficits throughout the Eighties.

Since health care costs now (through Medicare and Medicaid) significantly contributed to the deficit problem, the Reagan Administration soon became as interested in health care cost containment as their Democratic predecessors had been. With the support of a working majority in Congress, the Reagan Administration devised a two-pronged cost containment strategy that effectively accelerated the relative decline of physician and AMA power within health care.

The first element entailed efforts to foster competition in the sheltered health care industry (Melhado et al., 1988). The federal government worked to eliminate layers of health regulations and planning requirements that had been put in place during the previous fifteen years. They encouraged state governments to do likewise (for example, to eliminate Certificate of Need requirements for facilities construction). They also called on employers in both the private and public sectors to exercise their market power (the defacto control they have over the medical choices of their employees) to drive harder bargains with health providers.

In this new atmosphere, health care organizations themselves became more "corporatized" and economically-minded (Starr, 1982). The rise of health provider corporations (many of them for-profit) and the more general adoption of business practices that had long been standard in other economic sectors further reduced the professional power of physicians, and, inevitably, the AMA. To a greater and greater extent, physicians became employees, in fact if not in name (Jones, 1988). The hospitals and clinics that they worked in, as well as the insurance companies they billed through their practices, began to limit their cherished and traditional autonomy in fee-setting and diagnosis. Utilization review became customary, second opinions highly desirable or mandatory.

The second element in federal strategy involved more detailed and elaborate cost controls than had ever been employed before. Based upon a good deal of health economic theory, and experimental programs in New Jersey, the federal government moved in 1983 from a "cost-plus" to a prospective payment system (PPS) for Medicare (Kronenfeld and Whicker, 1984). Treatments were placed into specific Diagnosis Related Groups (DRGs), which in turn were linked to fixed governmental reimbursement. Health care facilities which provided treatment for less cost than the stated reimbursement could pocket the difference, while treatment costs over the stated limits became losses.

The prospective payment system placed tremendous pressure on health providers to reduce treatment inputs. Since much of this treatment is in fact prescribed by physicians (who were not directly controlled by the new legislation), the facilities now had clear incentives to reduce the use of physicians, and to control their behavior more closely when they were involved (Yaggy and Hodgson, 1985). The Medicare PPS thus drove a wedge into the physician hospital alliance of the Sixties and Seventies.

Initially, only Medicare payment was done through a PPS, but other payers rapidly adopted the federal government's (or a similar) system. The net effect was to decisively shift power within the health care system from providers to payers. This trend will continue with the adoption (as before, beginning with Medicare) of Resource-Based Relative Value Systems (RBRVS) for physician compensation in the 1990s. This latest system will bring about a greater standardization of physician charges. The already eroded discretionary power of doctors to set their own rates will be further weakened.

What Future for the AMA?

By the early Nineties, the physician-dominated system of health care, which the AMA had established seventy years before and vigorously defended ever since, was in tatters (Ginzberg, 1990). A continually-rising proportion of doctors were in salaried practice, many with Health Maintenance Organizations (HMOs) — the successors to the prepaid group practices that the AMA had fought so bitterly in the Thirties and Forties. It was not simply that the AMA had lost power. More fundamentally, the consensus definition of physician professionalism that the AMA had fostered through the "scientific medicine" movement was gone, probably forever. Now physicians were salaried as well as independently practicing. They worked in wider and wider ranges of specialties; including, ironically, family and general practice (Wagner, 1990). In urban areas, some widely advertised their services in newspapers and on television — behavior that some of the founders of the AMA would certainly find shameful and disgusting were they to witness it. Some enterprising doctors even owned their own hospitals, laboratories and clinics. They often became thriving business executives. But were they still physicians?

Elite groups facing the threat of long-term decay usually display the symptoms of identity loss, ideological dissension, group fragmentation and eroding self-confidence. The AMA itself is internally divided over future policy directions. Some elements are resigned to a continuation of present trends, and advocate more physician training in areas such as marketing and management. Others foresee eventual system breakdown, and the adoption of one or another form of national health insurance. (The editor of JAMA, George Lundberg, has stated as much, and devoted an entire 1991 issue of the Journal to examination of various national health insurance possibilities). Some conservative reformers would support a national health insurance system that preserved traditional physician roles (Holahan et al.; 1991). Other AMA physicians argue for unstinting opposition to any further governmental encroachment.

Ultimately, of course, the fate of the AMA, and the physician paradigm that it has always advanced, is at the mercy of larger events within the American health care system, and the society it operates within. AMA members are no more confused and divided over future directions in U.S. health care than other policymaking participants. Given the currently pervasive national skepticism and cynicism toward most aspects of public governance, how could it be otherwise? Given the enormous financial, ethical, clinical and legal problems stemming from such contemporary health care problems as AIDS, drug addiction, poverty, and "the graying of America", it would be astounding if any major health care interest group could develop and project a consistent and coherent policy vision at this time.

The American health care system is simultaneously experiencing great successes and major failures. "Scientific medicine" has produced notable triumphs in care, but at an unsustainable financial cost (Cooper, 1991). Some observers, including some physicians, still call for a return to the presumably more benign days in which health care and physician practice were separated from economics - health care as a mission, or a public service, rather than as a business. Given the problems that all current health care systems are having with cost control, access to care and quality improvement, this is escapist thinking.

As the U.S. health care sector and associated public policies advance into a new millenium, the issue of appropriate resource allocation will loom larger than ever before. The challenge health care professionals face is to invent a system that balance economic realities with clinical possibilities in an ethically acceptable manner. In this task, the examples provided by other nations may offer useful insights, but no real blueprints for the future.

The collected works in this book show that one organization was created to meet just such a challenge when it materialized in the 19th

Century. The American Medical Association has, more than any other organization, faced the nation's fundamental health care problems throughout history, and devised means of addressing them.

Some of their prescriptions may be fairly criticized as short-sighted, or self-interested. Others have clearly become obsolete with time. Nevertheless, over the last century, the movement for "scientific medicine" that the AMA spearheaded has resulted in immeasurable benefits for not only the U.S., but the world. The AMA has also proven that it can be a resilient and innovative organization when faced with the clear need for fundamental change.

With the urgent and critical choices that we face in designing a new health care system to meet changing needs, a renewed and revitalized American Medical Association would have a potentially important part to play. In a coalition with other social and medical groups, the AMA once helped invent an American health care system that met the needs of its time. Could it effectively do so again? Our health care future will be greatly affected by the answer to this question.

CHRONOLOGY

The following includes events directly related to the AMA and U.S. organized medicine, as well as other occurrences which had a substantial impact on health care and the AMA.

1760	New York City creates the first physician licensing laws requiring examination.
1765	The College of Physicians opens the nation's first medical school (now University of Pennsylvania). Rapid growth in schools from 1812 to 1906 (high point was 1902).
1766	New Jersey is the first province to begin a medical society. By the 1790's, several states begin authorizing state medical societies to license physicians with little positive effect. During the 1830's and 40's, licensing regresses until the late 1870's.

1797	The Medical Repository, a quarterly by New York editors, is the first Medical periodical in the U.S.
1798	U.S. Federal government starts special care for sick and disabled seamen; early beginnings of U.S. Public Health Service (so named in 1912).
1812	New England Journal of Medicine and Surgery is published.
1839	Flexible tube stethoscope is invented by Pennock.
1844	"Laughing gas" is used as an anesthesia. 1846 sees first surgery using anesthesia (ether).
1847	AMA is founded by an allopathic group, seeking professional self-regulation through medical ethics and actions to identify and limit quacks and cult practitioners such as the Thomsonians, Eclectics and Homeopaths.
1858	AMA's first Committee on Ethics is established.
1859	AMA creates six "Scientific Sections" as organizational elements to promote science.
1860's	Medical specialties first gain acceptance and initial growth.
1867	Joseph Lister introduces carbolic acid spray as an antisepsis for surgery. By the 1880's, sterilization through aseptic practice greatly reduces surgical mortality rates.
1869	Massachusetts forms first state board of health.
1870	Harvard's President Eliot reorganizes the Harvard Medical School, significantly raising standards, course and program duration, adding laboratories, and research. The University of Pennsylvania and others follow soon.

1870's	Rapid growth in hospitals occurs into 1920's. Causes include improved surgery, other technology and nursing.
1870's	Knowledge of bacteriology is promoted by Pasteur and Koch led to major advances in preventive medicine.
1873	Texas establishes first state board of medical examiners. A rapid surge in other states initiating licensing boards occurs in the 1880's and 90's.
1873	First nursing schools are established in Boston, New Haven and New York City.
1876	Twenty-two medical schools form the Association of American Medical Colleges.
1876	The American Public Health Association is founded as a voluntary organization.
1877	State of Illinois legislation limits licensing of physicians to graduates of approved medical schools, while requiring registration of all physicians.
1879	Congress establishes the National Board of Health. Their rating of medical schools uses evaluation criteria adopted by the AMA.
1883	The Journal of the American Medical Association (JAMA) is established.
1886	The Association of American Physicians splits off from the AMA as a group of scientific doctors with little patience for political, ethical and organizational activities.
1890	First national association of medical schools begins (Today's Association of American Medical Colleges).
1890's	Osteopathy, Chiropractic and Christian Science "sects" begin to challenge "regular scientific" medicine.

1891	The National Confederation of State Medical Examining and Licensing Boards is established.
1893	Johns Hopkins Medical School is founded, setting new standards such as college degree for preadmissions and four years of medical school as graduate study in scientific research and clinical instruction.
1895	The X-ray is introduced, adding to the fast increasing importance of hospitals.
1898	AMA's Committee on Scientific Research is established to provide grants for fostering medical research.
1899	AMA's Committee on National Legislation is created to represent the association's interests in Washington.
1899	AMA's Bureau of Exhibits is established to promote medical education.
1899	The Medical Library Association is founded.
1899	Association of Hospital Superintendents is founded in Cleveland, OH (now the American Hospital Association).
1899	Dr. Simmon begins a 25 years appointment as Editor of JAMA and develops the journal into an internationally recognized publication which also earns the lifeblood income to finance many AMA programs.
1901	The AMA reorganizes, creating the policy making House of Delegates with representation based on state and county societies. Membership in AMA would now hopefully consist of all members of local societies as affiliated with state societies. Membership increases tenfold by 1910. By the 1920's, many hospitals require physicians to be members of county medical societies before affiliation with hospital.

1902	AMA acquires its first permanent headquarters in Chicago.
1904	AMA establishes the Council on Medical Education to enhance and standardize requirements for medical schools.
1905	AMA establishes the Council on Pharmacy and Chemistry to set standards on drug manufacturing and advertising, and fight the war on quack prescriptions and the nostrum trade. The AMA Chemical Laboratory is established in 1906 to evaluate nostrums and drugs submitted for approval.
1906	Congress passes the Pure Food and Drug Act, beginning limited federal regulation.
1906	AMA's first American Medical Directory is published, listing over 128,000 physicians in the U.S. and Canada. Unlicensed physicians are excluded.
1907	AMA visits and evaluates all medical schools; report generates reforms.
1908	The AMA's Archives of Internal Medicine is published; counterpart specialty journals soon follow on pediatrics and surgery.
1910	The Flexner Report, funded by the Carnegie Foundation at the request of the AMA, is released. The report helps accelerate a systemic restructuring and new standards for medical schools. The report recommends closing all but 31 of 131 schools and improving those remaining. It cites many cases of diploma mills turning out excessive, poorly prepared doctors. Johns Hopkins is hailed as the model school. By 1915, 95 schools remain, many failing financially due to the increased licensing requirement standards by the states. Entry to the physician profession quickly becomes limited, while prestige and income soar over the next two decades.

1912	The Federation of State Medical Boards is established, accepting AMA's rating of medical schools as authoritative, making the AMA the de facto national accrediting agency for medical schools.
1912	Vitamin A is discovered.
1914	The AMA's Council on Medical Education sets standards for hospital intern programs and publishes first list of approved internship hospitals. It is redesignated the Council on Medical Education and Hospitals in 1920.
1914	Major cities receive pasteurized milk.
1915	The National Board of Medical Examiners is founded.
1916	AMA's Committee on Social Insurance recommends compulsory state health insurance. The Committee helps draft legislation in Massachusetts and New York with the Association for Labor Legislation.
1917	The American College of Surgeons begins their Hospital Standards Program; five minimum standards are adopted in 1919.
1917	Ophthalmology establishes the first national specialty board for certification. Medical specialization grows rapidly. Nursing and allied health personnel also quickly increase.
1920	AMA opposes compulsory health insurance through an August 1920 resolution by the House of Delegates.
1921	AMA opposes group medical practice and contract practice.
1922	Insulin is discovered as a treatment for diabetes.
1922	The Woman's Auxiliary to the AMA is established for "wives of doctors," as an outgrowth of state and county auxiliaries.

1924	AMA's Council on Medical Education and Hospitals begin approving hospitals for residency specialty training.
1924	Dr. Morris Fishbein becomes Editor of the JAMA and quickly leads the war against "socialized medicine."
1925	AMA's Council on Physical Medicine is established to evaluate devices sold for diagnostic and therapeutic uses, e.g., ultraviolet radiation, hearing aids and artificial limbs.
1928	Penicillin is discovered by Fleming, permitting antibiotic therapy.
1929	Baylor University Hospital in Dallas starts the first major medical insurance program for school teachers. Blue Cross and Blue Shield, as well as commercial insurers proliferate in the 1930s and 40s. Health care quickly becomes big business.
1930	The National Institute of Health is founded to promote medical research.
1930's	Many "wonder Drugs" like sulfa, penicillin and streptomycin are released.
1931	The electronic microscope is discovered.
1931	AMA's Bureau of Medical Economics is established.
1932	AMA opposes prepayment plans such as Blue Cross.
1932	The final report of the Committee on the Costs of Medical Care recommends government intervention, payment of medical care through taxation, and greater use of group practice to remedy shortfalls in care to the poor.
1935	Social Security Act is approved on August 14. It does not include compulsory health insurance due to AMA influence.

1935	The California State Medical Society unsuccessfully submits legislation calling for compulsory and voluntary health insurance.
1936	AMA's Council on Foods (later: Foods and Nutrition) becomes independent from the Council on Pharmacy and Chemistry.
1937	AMA advocates county medical societies to help share the burden of caring for indigent patients.
1937	The National Cancer Institute is established as the first national medical specialty center.
1937	First blood bank is established by Cook County, Illinois.
1938	Congress adopts a substantially stronger Food, Drug and Cosmetic Act.
1939	Senator Robert Wagner (Dem/NY) introduces a national health bill as part of Social Security; does not pass Committees.
1940s	WWII creates the demand for extensive medical research and training of new physicians. The GI Bill funds much of the training.
1943	The Wagner-Murray-Dingell bill for comprehensive health insurance under Social Security is introduced in Congress but no action was taken.
1944	President Roosevelt's State of the Union Speech calls for the right to adequate medical care as part of an economic bill of rights.
1945	President Truman proposes a national health insurance (NHI) program for all Americans, in addition to more federal money for research and hospital construction. A revised Wagner-Murray-Dingell bill is introduced. AMA fights NHI.
1946	The Hospital Survey and Construction Act (Hill-Burton) is passed in Congress.

1947	American Academy of Family Physicians is founded.
1947	The Wagner-Murray-Dingell bill is re-introduced.
1948	AMA hires Whittaker and Baxter, a California Public Relations Firm, to work a campaign against Truman's plan for national health insurance.
1950	The Social Security Act is amended to provide for direct payments to hospitals and doctors by the States, with federal matching funds.
1951	The Joint Commission on Accreditation of Hospitals is formed by the American College of Surgeons, American College of Physicians, American Hospital Association, AMA and the Canadian Medical Association.
1952	First open-heart operation. DNA identified with genetics.
1952	The Murray-Humphrey-Dingell-Celler bills for health insurance for social security beneficiaries are introduced to Congress.
1953	U.S. government establishes the Department of Health, Education and Welfare (now HHS).
1955	Salk polio vaccine is available.
1957	The Forand bill calling for health insurance for social security beneficiaries is introduced into Congress. It was reintroduced unsuccessfully in 1959.
1960	The Kennedy-Anderson bill calling for an expanded Forand bill is unsuccessfully introduced and again in 1961, and (as Medicare) in 1963, 1964, and 1965. The Kerr-Mills bill is passed, providing matching federal and state aid for the poor.
1961	The AMA forms the American Medical Political Action Committee to fight national health care legislation.

1965	The Mill's Medicare Bill is substituted for the King-Anderson Bill and finally passes in July.
1966	AMA publishes its report on internship and residency training in *The Graduate Education of Physicians.*
1971	National Cancer Act begins the crusade against cancer.
1972	HMO Act.
1975	AMA streamlines its organization and begins recovery efforts to strengthen membership and resources, better represent specialty groups, and make their political lobby more proactive.
1975-1989	Defeat of Carter Hospital Cost Legislation--Introduction of Medicare PPS
1989	American Medical Television begins.
1989	New AMA headquarters building opens in Chicago.
1991	AMA proposes reform of the U.S. health care system (Health Access America) to include expansion of health insurance coverage.
1992	Health Care costs U.S. citizens nearly $2 billion a day, as the nation's biggest business and number two employer (behind education).

2

THE STATUS OF MEDICINE IN THE MID-NINETEENTH CENTURY

Like the United States in general, American medicine in the middle of the nineteenth century was characterized by disorganization and decentralization in structure, and extreme entrepreneurism and individualism in practice. There were only a handful of universities engaging in significant medical and scientific research. Consequently, the level of clinical development in American health care lagged behind that seen in major European centers such as London, Paris and Vienna. While many U.S. physicians were happy to adopt medical advances developed in the Old World, the difficulties in communicating across a vast ocean in the pre-electronic era ensured that news of such developments would be received after a long time period–if at all.

Authors in this section chronicle the fascinating, colorful and often horrifying results of largely prescientific American medicine. Given the lack of knowledge of basic principles of antisepsis and sanitation, as well as the relatively primitive level of technological development in areas such as surgery and anesthesia, medical procedures were often ineffective and painful. Hospitals were grim facilities that were more often thought of as places of death rather than recovery. Anyone with the money for it preferred home treatment, or (if wealthy and the condition sufficiently serious) a trip to Europe for the best care available. Those who had no real choice–Union and Confederate soldiers wounded during the Civil War, for example–often found that quick death on the battlefield was preferable to the lingering miseries imposed by the painful and inexpert care of military surgeons.

The general status and public perceptions of medical education and physicians reflected this state of underdevelopment. Readings here point out that there was no standard educational curriculum. While a large number of medical schools tried their best to provide adequate training, all too many were ill-equipped and staffed fly-by-night entities which emphasized profit-making over instructional soundness. In such institutions, students learned what they could from available faculty (sometimes practicing their skills on cadavers obtained through grave-robbing), and then left after some time period (from 3 - 4 months to two years) calling themselves "doctors".

Protection from unqualified medical practitioners was slight at best, since physician licensing standards (handled, then as now, at the state level) were often minimal to nonexistent. Where licensing procedures did have some value, as in Massachusetts, South Carolina, Maryland and Ohio, they were often used by one group of physicians to punish another during periodic outbreaks of bitter conflict over clinical and professional practices. These conflicts were to some extent an inevitable byproduct of a developing medical profession that lacked a sound professional identity. Medical practice ethics were borrowed from the principles set down by European physicians (most prominently, Percival's writings from England), but no effective enforcement mechanism existed. Even if publicly exposed, dishonest and incompetent doctors usually continued their practices after moving to a new location.

Not surprisingly, the average citizen regarded physicians with suspicion. Physicians often received very low compensation for their services, living and practicing in threadbare and often squalid conditions. In a society characterized by Jacksonian democracy and the primacy of the individual, a wide variety of health movements ("cults", to their detractors) flourished, often with charismatic leaders. Authors here outline the activities of such sectarians as Samuel Thomson and Mary Baker Eddy. These sects reflected broader sociopolitical interests (such as vegetarianism and feminism) as well as popular dissatisfaction with the quality of available medical care.

As with other areas of American economic activity, health care was characterized by laissez-faire principles of small business capitalism. An American citizen could select from doctors professing allegiance to a wide range of scientific and philosophical theories for his or her treatment. The dark side of this diversity and flexibility could be summed up by the phrase "caveat emptor"--let the buyer beware. There were no real regulatory protections for the patient. Nor were prescriptions needed to obtain pharmaceuticals. Not surprisingly, medical quacks often thrived. Their nostrums, along with high rates of self-medication, led to widespread poisoning and drug addiction rates far beyond those seen today.

Although states varied in their supervision of medical practices within their borders, none in the 1800s took on the broad responsibility for consumer protection routinely assumed today. The Federal Government did not involve itself at all with health care matters, except in limited areas of relevance (the qualifications of physicians practicing in the Army and Navy, for example). Major efforts to change the nature of medical regulation, education and practice therefore had to come from health care practitioners themselves.

The health care reform movement began at the state and local levels. Its proponents had concluded that the current structure of health care in the U.S. was totally inadequate (even the existing patchwork of licensure was disintegrating under prolonged assaults at the state level). Primarily directed by physicians from their state and local medical societies, the motivation was two-fold: to make American health care more scientific and reliable, and to improve the economic well-being of "real" physicians (allopaths--the "sects" and homeopaths would have to go). Historical accounts that emphasize one or the other concern provide a misleading picture. The physicians that tried to change American health care wanted to both do well *and* do good.

By the 1840s, the basic tenets of the reform movement were firmly established:

1) Medical education would have to be thoroughly overhauled and standardized along "scientific" lines. Medical schools should be modeled after the best European institutions, with a research component and access to hospital facilities.

2) Attempts to practice "unsound" or "unscientific" medicine would have to be precluded by government regulations (especially licensure laws) at the national and/or state levels. Medical quackery and sectarianism must be criminalized, not tolerated as unconventional treatment.

3) The public would have to be educated to the necessity of such a system of health care. This education would become part of the larger public health movement, which called for improved hygiene and sanitation.

4) The "destructive" laissez-faire competition between small businessmen/physicians would have to end, since scientifically- trained physicians could not function properly

in an unfettered marketplace. Physicians would have to be permitted to maintain dignified and publicly respected--and lucrative--practices. Once again, government regulations (on advertising and solicitation, among other things) would be used to enforce this state of affairs.

Orthodox physicians favoring these reform principles gradually extended their coalition-building beyond the state level. In 1846, they held their first national conference in New York. In 1847, at their second meeting, they formally named their collectivity the "American Medical Association". Though its initial impact would be quite modest, the organization that would radically change the role of the physician in American health care was finally established.

(A) Books

1. Bordley, James and Harvey A. McGhee. *Two Centuries of American Medicine, 1776-1976.* Philadelphia: W. B. Saunders, 1976.

This is an outstanding historical account of the advances in medical education and the prevention and treatment of disease in the first two centuries of the American state. The book begins with a description of the primitive treatment regimen given George Washington in the last twenty-four hours of his life and takes us through the many developments that have taken place since. There is a comprehensive chapter on the AMA and numerous sections relating the rise of organized medicine to other events in the society. The authors have compiled many insightful cartoons, photographs, tables, and excerpts from popular literature that enhances the text as a historical document.

2. Gevitz, Norman. *The D.O.'s: Osteopathic Medicine in America.* Baltimore, MD: The Johns Hopkins University Press, 1982.

Gevitz' book provides the first comprehensive portrait of the osteopathic medical profession in the U.S. He traces the many developments from the late nineteenth century through today. Included in his analysis are discussions of the many leaders of the osteopathic movement and the ideas and institutions that shaped the profession. Changes in the belief system, educational programs, and scope of practice are addressed against the backdrop of parallel developments in allopathic medicine.

The relationship between osteopaths and the AMA has been a tumultuous one, most notably in the 1940's when Morris Fishbein, editor of JAMA, referred to osteopaths as "cultists" and participated in an AMA movement designed to assure that the American Association of Medical Colleges would not allow osteopathic programs to award M.D. degrees. However in the 1950's, under the leadership of John W. Cline, the AMA began to accept osteopathy's legitimacy and even conducted studies and "inspections" that concluded that much of the old "cultist" stigma and non-medical beliefs of osteopathy had dissipated. The newer view of osteopathic education was that it would suffice in the training of general practitioners. As the profession of osteopathic medicine grew the AMA began to take another look. In the 1960's, according to Gevitz, the AMA adopted a series of new resolutions aimed at destroying the American Osteopathic Association (AOA). The AMA, it seems, planned to absorb the osteopathic profession, its schools and AOA members "quickly, before organized osteopathy became too powerful" (p. 124). These efforts failed and the AOA remained intact as a professional association. Since those days of struggle the osteopathic medical profession, according to the author, "is now growing so rapidly and making such a significant contribution to American health care that it can no longer be ignored" (p. 147).

3. Kaufman, Martin. *American Medical Education: The Formative Years, 1765-1910.* Westport, CT: Greenwood Press, 1976.

Despite the title, the author describes the book to be not a history of U.S. medical education, but instead "an examination of the major trends and developments that affected the colleges" (p. ix). This distinction is subtle at best, since the book is a short (less than 200 pages) and rather straightforward chronology. Its eleven chapters cover the development of American medical education from its colonial beginnings up to the impact of the Flexner Report in the first decade after its release. In addition to the usual secondary sources, Kaufman utilizes a wide variety of collections of private papers (including those of Abraham Flexner), and official records and documents.

From the available evidence, Kaufman begins his account by emphasizing the challenges faced in a rugged and inhospitable New World by the few physicians who were willing to leave Europe. At times, their efforts to provide additional physicians through primitive educational programs met with great public disapproval. (In 1788, for example, New Yorkers rioted and assaulted a group of medical students and professors; they had engaged in habitual grave-robbing to replenish their supply of cadavers, and would occasionally hang a body part or two out of a window to attract public attention.) From here, American medical education went downhill until the mid 1800's.

Despite the founding of the American Medical Association in 1847, and some state-level attempts at reform, Kaufman emphasizes the uneven development of U.S. physician training and practice until the twentieth century (not least, with chapter titles such as "The Situation Deteriorates Further, 1860-1890," and "Sporadic Improvements"). In Kaufman's opinion, the crucial turning point came with the establishment of Johns Hopkins University, and the selection of Daniel Coit Gilman (then-President of the University of California) as the first President. Johns Hopkins, with a large endowment, did not have to rely upon student fees to remain viable, and Gilman organized its medical curriculum according to the most European principles (primarily German).

With Johns Hopkins as its center, the medical reform movement redoubled its efforts. Kaufman briefly describes the efforts of the Council on Medical Education and the Association of American Medical Colleges, and how they led to the Carnegie Foundation's commission of the landmark study by Abraham Flexner analyzing the state of American physician training. The enormous impact of the Flexner Report on American medicine is outlined in the final chapter of the book, but (as with other topics) very briefly.

The virtues and defects of this work stem from the decision of the author to provide a short description of the major events in American medical education over a 140-year period. Anyone wishing to get a capsule summary of how U.S. physician training got to its current state will find this book handy. At the same time, however, it necessarily skims the surface of complex events and patterns of development that require much more detailed (and deeper) treatment for complete understanding.

In addition, Kaufman does not attempt to provide the reader with any sense of the greater significance of the events that he describes, or any but the briefest connections between the developments in American medical education and simultaneous social, economic and political changes in the nation as a whole. He develops an uncomplicated and focused historical narrative, and leaves it at that.

4. Kett, Joseph F. *The Formation of the Medical Profession.* New Haven, CT: Yale University Press, 1968.

In this short book (180 pages of text), Joseph Kett chronicles the development of medical training and practice in the United States between 1780 and 1860, focusing on the topics of licensure, organization, education and sectarianism. (The book itself is a revised version of Dr. Kett's Ph.D. thesis at Yale.) While agreeing with the great majority of historians that nineteenth century health care standards in America were uneven and generally poor, the author argues that informal practices and voluntary action mitigated some of the worst results of a medical profession that did not have effective national methods of enforcing standards of quality. As appendices, the author includes a summary of licensing legislation and a discussion of "irregular practitioners in the United States".

The first of the book's six chapters describes "the weak arm of the law" and the wide range of medical behavior that resulted in both the U.S. and England from the Seventeenth through mid-nineteenth centuries. The lack of anything approaching uniform expectations in medical knowledge and behavior was a prolific source of discord (Chapter 2). In particular, there was continual conflict between universities, which argued that medical degrees from their institutions should be considered practicing licenses, and private professional societies which vigorously disagreed. Chapter 3, "The Perils of Control," outlines the legal and professional problems that resulted in states such as Massachusetts, South Carolina, Maryland and Ohio whenever one group or another gained the ability to punish its rivals through the use of state regulations. Given the lack of consensus over standards, or even the very definition of proper medical practice, it is not surprising that various "sects" rose with radical visions of care and healing. Kett describes the careers of such notable sectarians as Samuel Thomson and Elisha Perkins, showing how their eccentric medical theories fit into wider sociopolitical concerns of the time, such as antimonopolism and feminism (Chapter 4).

In similar fashion, Chapter 5 covers "Homeopathy and Its Kindred Delusions," including such diverse phenomena as mesmerism, phrenology and Swedenborgianism. Gradually, however, more orthodox doctors, wishing to base clinical practice on the scientific principles developing in European medicine, decided to engage in wider organization and coalition-building. Galvanized by the repeal of licensure laws in several states, a number of these physicians called a national medical convention in New York in 1846. At their third annual meeting in 1848, they declared themselves to be the "American Medical Association".

In the concluding chapter of the book, Kett discusses their activities up until 1860. The author concludes that while "intended as an agency of reform, the Association was in fact a microcosm of the profession and reflected all its weaknesses" (p. 173). Though the tide was gradually turning in favor of scientific medicine, its final triumph would not come for another half-century.

5. Ludmerer, Kenneth M. *Learning to Heal.* New York: Basic Books, Inc., 1985.

Subtitled "The Development of American Medical Education," this book provides a chronology from the mid-nineteenth Century to the present. The 280 text pages are divided into fourteen chapters. The author is a Professor in the Departments of History and Internal Medicine at Washington University in St. Louis.

The author begins by stating that "contrary to popular perception, neither Abraham Flexner nor the American Medical Association participated in the creation of modern American medical education. Both played important roles in its later development, but by that time the conceptual revolution in how medicine should be taught had already taken place and the university medical school had already appeared. Nevertheless, both Flexner and the AMA profoundly influenced the final form that the system took" (p.7)--research-oriented and university based. When fundamental educational reforms did take place at the most innovative medical schools (Harvard and Pennsylvania, for example) the AMA took credit for influence that it did not in fact have over these institutions. As Dr. Ludmerer points out, the AMA pushed vigorously for reforms of U.S. medical education, but had little success during the 19th Century.

By 1910, the AMA's influence had indeed increased. But the medical education proposals it advocated had originated in the most advanced medical schools. The AMA Council on Medical Education was in fact staffed with and controlled by medical educators, and served primarily to disseminate ideas that had been developed elsewhere. Medical practitioners, not academics, were the primary audience for AMA guidance on the issues of the day. In contrast, "academic physicians were much more closely identified with the AAMC and the various medical research societies" (p.129). Ironically, though, the AMA and its members were major beneficiaries of the enhanced social prestige and influence that resulted from the greater effectiveness of medical education.

After 1910, the AMA's greatest contribution to medical education reform came in the area of political action. Through the Association's influence over state medical boards, it could determine whether a given medical school's diploma would be accepted or not. Consequently, medical schools hastened to conform with the AMA guidelines in their curricula and instruction. The medical school rating by the AMA Council on Medical Education became authoritative for the National Board of Medical Examiners, and unapproved schools were forced to close.

Dr. Ludmerer concludes that "the AMA's role in the development of American medical education is long overdue for critical evaluation"

(p. 238). The Association had almost no impact in the 19th Century, and its role in the 20th was largely one of facilitating the adoption of reforms that others had devised. This latter aspect of AMA activity was, however, critically important. Particularly in the area of state licensing, the AMA played a part "that was profound, even if much more circumscribed than commonly realized" (p. 240).

6. Marti-Ibanez, Felix, Editor. *History of American Medicine.* New York, NY: MD Publications, Inc., 1959.

This is a symposium dealing with various aspects of American medical history. Its editor is Professor and Director of the Department of the History of Medicine at New York Medical College. The symposium was previously published in the International Record of Medicine, and is reproduced as one in a series of medical symposia by MD Publications, Inc. The text, running about 175 pages, contains fourteen essays. Many focus on the varied state of American medical care in the eighteenth and nineteenth centuries ("Medicine and Medical Practices among Aboriginal American Indians," "Diseases and Medical Practice in Colonial America," and "Medical Education and Medical Schools in Colonial America"). Others ("The Evolution of Medical Research in the United States") cover more up-to-date developments. In "A Brief Sketch of the Rise of American Medical Societies," W. B. McDaniel II portrays American physicians as "the most completely organized of all the professions. At the apex is a national association of our physicians—the American Medical Association" (p. 133).

7. Norwood, W. F. *Medical Education in the United States Before the Civil War.* Philadelphia, PA: University of Pennsylvania Press, 1944.

This book focuses on the rise and progress of medical education only up to the Civil War looking at some of the smaller, lesser-known medical schools. Up until the Civil War medical education gave very little to the world. The generally accepted method of medical instruction was the preceptorship. And standards of instruction were obviously in the hands of the preceptor.

Establishment of early medical schools did little to help these shortcomings. Many of the schools of the mid-1800s had not concerned themselves with educational ethics, but began to adopt the code of the young American Medical Association (AMA). It was actually the effort to raise the standards of medical education that brought about the founding of the AMA.

In 1849, the founder of the AMA, N. S. Davis, pointed out four faults that contributed to the uncertainty of medical science: " (1) the American trait exhibited by an urge to rush everything in a hurry; (2) the almost universal neglect of proper preliminary education; (3) the defective organization of most of the numerous medical schools; and (4) the inordinate expense of a medical education." AMA reforms advocated lengthening school terms, increasing professorships, examinations conducted by impartial persons, and standardized pre-medical education. Although initial response to the AMA reforms was limited, the course medical education later followed, was the format suggested by the AMA.

8. Shafer, Henry Burnell. *The American Medical Profession 1783-1850*. New York, NY: AMS Press, 1968.

This work is a reprint of a 1936 edition that was produced by Columbia University Press as part of their Studies in the Social Sciences series. The book consists of a preface, eight chapters (almost 250 text pages), a bibliographical note and an index. After an initial survey chapter, the narrative is topic-centered, with a straightforward chronology within each chapter. Chapter topics include "Medical Education," "The Practice of Physics," "Medical Ethics and Fees," "Medical Literature" and "Medical Regulations and Societies."

As might be expected, most of the book is devoted to the evolution of the physician profession in the U.S. before the establishment of the American Medical Association. Within each chapter, there is brief coverage of AMA activities in the relevant area. In "Medical Education," Dr. Shafer emphasizes that the influence of the AMA was limited, given its fledgling status and reliance upon voluntary acceptance of its recommendations. The Association gathered data, and a committee chaired by Nathan Smith Davis recommended that local medical societies have the right to examine students and to expel unqualified physicians. Between 1848 and 1850, the AMA adopted a number of resolutions concerning educational reform. According to the author, this work "did bring to national attention the state of education and the need for reform, and furnished a valuable forum for discussion" (p. 95).

In "Medical Ethics and Fees," the author mentions that the AMA incorporated Percival's principles into its code of medical ethics. This was not an isolated instance of borrowing; Dr. Shafer claims in "Medical Literature" that "much of the work of American medical writers consisted in editing work of British authors, a fact admitted by the American Medical Association in its report of 1848" (p. 178).

In "Medical Regulations and Societies," the various reform positions of the AMA are briefly mentioned in passing (temperance and the adoption of pure food and drug legislation, for example). At the conclusion of the chapter, Dr. Shafer provides a short account of the formation of the AMA, pointing out that "lack of interest in the local societies delayed the formation of a national association. . . until 1846" (p. 237). Once formed, however, the AMA would provide "a national agency through which reforms and ideas could be nationalized" (p. 240).

9. Shryock, Richard H. "Medical Licensing in America, 1650-1965." Baltimore: Johns Hopkins Press, 1957.

In his second book on American medicine, Professor Shryock traces licensing for physicians from its pre-regulated stage he calls "Early Licensing and Subsequent Decadence." He goes on to describe an extended period of reform beginning in the late 1800's and lasting on into the 1960's. One culminating event of the reform period described by the author was a 1961 conference sponsored by the AMA and the Food and Drug Administration. The title of the conference is telling, "National Congress on Medical Quackery" offered presumably to educate both Congress and the public. Following this the public began to scrutinize medical practice more than ever before with popular articles appearing in *Life*, *Look*, *The Atlantic*, and the *New Yorker* for the first time. Licensure came to be seen as only part of the answer for assuring "good medical care." The author concludes his book with a look at the myriad problems associated with medical licensure.

10. Shryock, Richard H. "Medicine and Society in America, 1660-1860. " New York: New York University Press, 1960.

This book traces the development of organized medicine in American society from the mid-17th century to the mid-19th century. Professor Shryock approaches his analysis of this development from three perspectives: 1) medical thought and practice; 2) health and disease; and 3) medicine and society. In his expose on medical thought and practice there is a thorough accounting of the evolution of medicine's link to science and the emergence of hospitals as centers of technology and practice. The section on health and disease traces the epidemiological pattern of illness and the shift towards disease oriented treatment as defining the "medical model." Lastly, the author places the development of the medical profession in a larger social context. In this chapter the political climate of the mid 1800's is described by the author as Jacksonian Democracy proclaiming "inalienable rights to life, liberty, and quackery" (p. 149). From this environment, the AMA emerged as a loosely organized group of representatives of medical schools and state societies. "Its prime purpose was the reform of medical education, but it also hoped to encourage research, improve public health, and raise the level of professional ethics." (p. 149). Consistent with this mission, the newly formed AMA and the American Statistical Society were asked by Congress in 1850 to look at the relationship between disease and poverty in American cities. These findings, the author claims, led to the profound understanding "that gradual improvement in living conditions was a major influence, in the last analysis, in making for a similarly gradual increase in the life prospects of average individuals" (p. 166). Thus the AMA had made a major first contribution in raising the health status of the American people.

11. Shryock, Richard H. *Medicine in America, Historical Essay.* Baltimore, MD: The Johns Hopkins Press, 1966.

Medicine in America is a collection of historical essays, written between 1930 and 1962. Fifteen essays are arranged into six broad categories: "Period Pieces," "Personal and Public Hygiene," "The Medical Profession," "Medical Thought and Research," and "Historiography." There is also an introductory essay, "The Medical History of the American People." In the first essay, the American Medical Association is described as a force for reform. The development of the AMA Council on Medical Education in 1904 is briefly described. The production of the Flexner Report, along with the AMA participation in the establishment of the Federation of State Medical Boards and the Association of American Medical Colleges, are considered integral parts of what Dr. Shryock calls "the great turning point in the history of American medicine" (p. 32). AMA-supported government "pure food and drug" statutes are also numbered among the positive aspects of AMA activities. The strong AMA opposition to national health insurance is also mentioned, but the author feels that the Association will cooperate with "the first step toward a general adoption of compulsory insurance" (p. 45)--Medicare.

In "Medical Practice in the Old South," Dr. Shryock mentions that a number of leading Southern physicians participated in the founding and early operation of the AMA, despite growing Southern fears in the 1840s and 1850s of growing dependence on the North. However, the 1850s saw growing North-South tensions in the AMA as well as other national organizations.

AMA involvement in public health issues is covered in "The Early Public Health Movement." In 1848, the AMA recommended that state and local medical societies work with their states toward the upgrading of public health recordkeeping, and that "sanitary reform" be vigorously promoted. However, AMA public health activities were inadequate in the eyes of a number of physicians, who went on to found the American Public Health Association.

"The Medical Profession" covers the motivation for educational reform that was present in the founding of the AMA, as well as the difficulties the organization faced in getting its ideas accepted. The AMA efforts to control professional behavior through its Code of Ethics is mentioned. As Dr. Shryock points out, "they have since been criticized as providing 'trade union rules' or 'books of etiquette' rather than true ethics" (p. 157).

The author, in "Medical Sources and the Social Historian," suggests that on occasion the AMA has made valuable contributions to social history. Reports by the AMA's committee on hygiene in 1848 and 1849 "contain some of the first critical descriptions of slum conditions in growing American cities" (p. 291). In addition, "there are few more enlightening essays on the status of American culture than the reports on American medical literature submitted to the American Medical Association between 1848 and 1852" (p. 294).

(B) Articles

12. Blackstone, Erwin A. "The AMA and the Osteopaths: A Study of the Power of Organized Medicine." *The Antitrust Bulletin,* (1976): 405-440.

The author, as Professor of Economics at Temple University, presents a case for holding the AMA in violation of U.S. Anti-Trust laws for its attempts to exclude osteopaths from competing with M.D. physicians (allopaths.) Blackstone traces this battle from its roots in the 19th century and takes special efforts to show that AMA's actions were motivated primarily by economic factors rather than to ensure quality care medical practice. The author reviews AMA activities in licensing, medical schools, intern programs, government Medicaid reimbursements, federal aid for medical schools, and consultation arrangements.

Blackstone believes the main threat to M.D.s' came from the fact that osteopaths were quick to fill the need for general practice care as more and more allopaths chose to enter medical specialties. He concludes by suggesting that the continued separation between osteopaths and allopaths is beneficial to the public as a check to the power of organized medicine (AMA) and creator of desirable competition.

3

ESTABLISHING THE AMERICAN MEDICAL ASSOCIATION (1847-1901)

Medical science and clinical practice began to advance rapidly around the middle of the 19th Century. Louis Pasteur and others revolutionized the understanding of disease causation and prevention. Diverse practitioners (Joseph Lister, Florence Nightingale, and others) contributed to a growing sophistication in the methods of treatment and rehabilitation. With the advent of new and useful procedures and technologies in medicine, the potential to develop and implement a truly scientific model of health care was greater than ever before. These developments reinforced the efforts by U.S. doctors to bring the nation's medical system up to world-class standards.

Physician efforts to upgrade American medicine--and their own status--began with state medical society efforts. A reform coalition brought delegates together from a number of states in 1846 for an initial national conference. Reformers led by a New York State Medical Society member, Nathan Smith Davis, established a national association of doctors the following year. The American Medical Association delegates adopted a charter which emphasized the need for medical education reform. This meant clinical instruction, formal linkages between hospitals and medical schools, and much more stringent examination and licensure standards for aspiring doctors. A Code of Ethics, modeled after Percival's principles, was adopted as the model for all physicians to follow. (Some, however, argued that the "ethical principles" contained in the Code were in fact merely tenets of professional courtesy).

The newly-formed AMA was also determined to eliminate the medical "cults". The homeopaths were particular targets of the

AMA's wrath; not only were they "unscientific", but many were more affluent than the allopaths that made up the Association's rank and file. In the years to come, the Association would try to eliminate the homeopathic influence using almost every conceivable means at its disposal. When AMA members in New York Medical Society arranged a truce, the national leadership, enraged, responded by expelling the entire Society!

Despite vigorous efforts, however, the AMA met with little initial success in persuading state legislatures to adopt laws that would enforce their prescriptions. Association membership drives met with only modest success. And some groups were simply not welcome; the AMA excluded black and female physicians. Bitter factional disputes (particularly over the Code of Ethics) distracted the organization from its central mission. Opposition to the AMA agenda from many proprietary medical schools led to the exclusion of their representatives from the AMA national meeting in 1874. Disgusted with the infighting, a group of research - oriented physicians split off to form the Association of American Physicians in 1886. More generally, the disorganization and decentralization of American health care militated against reform efforts from any quarter. As with other interest groups, the activities of the AMA were disrupted in the 1860s by the Civil War and its aftermath. (There were no National Conferences during 1861 and 1862, and those held in subsequent war years lacked extensive representation of Southern physicians.) The general public, concerned with settlement and economic development of a vast continent, did not feel a sense of urgency about the issue. The diversity of medical practice that the AMA saw as threatening was in fact preferred by the vast majority of the American public at the time. Nor was there a consensus for reform within the medical profession. The large number of medical schools that had a financial stake in maintaining the existing lack of uniformity were usually able to forestall AMA efforts to promote state reform legislation. In 1876, when the Association of American Medical Colleges was established, disagreement over whether and how to change medical education standards virtually paralyzed the organization.

The AMA did gain some measure of success in the latter half of the 19th Century. There was a gradual upgrading of medical education throughout the U.S. In particular, the founding of the Johns Hopkins Hospital in Baltimore, Maryland brought world - class medicine to the public's attention. In 1871, the AMA had recommended a four - year curriculum for all medical schools. In 1891, Harvard Medical School adopted such a program. Founded in 1893, Johns Hopkins' Medical School followed the format. It would serve as the basic model for twentieth century medical education. Other organizations with similar interests developed in health care, including the Medical Library

Association and the Association of Hospital Superintendents in 1899. During this time period, the organizational structure of the Association steadily developed. In 1858, the AMA Committee on Ethics was set up, and the following year saw the formation of six "scientific sections" to promote the development and use of science in health care. The Association inaugurated its own *Journal* in 1883, to the general approval of the medical community. The launching of AMA's Council on Medical Education was perhaps the most significant step it would take in its drive for higher educational standards. To further promote medical education, the organization put together a Bureau of Exhibits in 1899. The Committee on Scientific Research was established in 1898 to provide grants for medical research.

The growing public health movement, centered in the major cities that were experiencing a major influx of immigrants from Southern and Eastern Europe, raised public awareness of the need for upgraded health standards and government regulation. States began to develop a more activist stance. In 1873, for example, Texas established the first state board of medical examiners. Most other states would follow in the 1880s and 1890s. In 1877, Illinois passed legislation that limited physician licensure to graduates of approved medical schools, and required registration of all physicians. It was not until 1869 that the first state board of health was founded (Massachusetts), but by 1900, *every* state had one. In 1876, the American Public Health Association was founded. The AMA was an active participant in movements for pure food and drug laws, school hygiene, vaccination, control of venereal disease, health recordkeeping (including disease reporting requirements for physicians), and (naturally) an end to dangerous and deceptive medical "quackery". The nation was dramatically changing. Rapid industrialization and technological change were bringing about the need for a more active governmental presence on a variety of fronts. AMA members wanted professional autonomy, and instinctively distrusted the rambunctious politics of their era. Yet they concluded--as most interest groups have that their *private* aspirations could only be attained through the use of *public* institutions--in particular, state and national regulatory agencies. The growing political sophistication and activism of the AMA was evidenced in 1899 by the establishment of a Committee on National Legislation to represent the organization's policy preferences before Congress.

As Burrow (1963) notes, the American Medical Association really assumed its current organizational form and functioning in 1901. At that year's conference, the Association adopted sweeping reforms. It created a House of Delegates, based on representation from state and county societies, to create Association policies. This provided a clear and tight link between the AMA and the state and local societies. The resulting organizational efficiency and effectiveness would serve the

Association well in the national political struggles to come. The stage was set for the American Medical Association to assume primary control over the development of American health care.

(A) Books

13. Burrow, James G. *AMA: Voice of American Medicine.* Baltimore, MD: Johns Hopkins Press, 1963.

In the Preface, James G. Burrow states his intention to provide a detailed and focused study of the development and evolution of the American Medical Association as a political force. While not an officially commissioned study, the author did receive significant assistance from the AMA staff at its Chicago headquarters. Nevertheless, Burrow declares that "the present volume embodies the results of independent investigation and makes no attempt to espouse the particular interest of any group" (p. v). At approximately four hundred pages in length, the study is a reasonably comprehensive political and social history.

Beginning with the establishment of the American Medical Association in 1847, the eighteen chapters follow the gradual expansion of the organization's political power and activism, culminating with the beginnings of the epic battle between the AMA-led conservative coalition in Congress and the Kennedy Administration (with its liberal/labor allies) over what would become Medicare and Medicaid in the Sixties. Since the book is undeniably dated (published in 1963), it is of limited use for researchers interested in understanding the current political activities of the AMA. Given that limitation, Burrow provides the reader with a well-researched and clearly written description of how the AMA has significantly helped to shape American health policy through political action. All of the major historical controversies that a reader would expect in such a work (the Pure Food and Drugs Act, the Wagner-Murray-Dingell bills, the Truman proposals for national health insurance, and so forth) are covered at length. Burrow analyzes each development with a high degree of scholarly objectivity and detachment. To his credit, Burrow also makes great efforts to describe how the political efforts of the AMA were in turn related to the overall transformation of the United States. Since the formation of the AMA, the U.S. has moved from a limited government industrial state into the largest economy in the world, with numerous but often unconnected welfare state components. It also has potentially dangerous social divisions (particularly those related to race) that detract from the overall effectiveness of the health care system.

One of Burrow's central points is that any attempt to classify the AMA as a purely "reactionary" or "status quo" political force is misguided and hopelessly simplistic. Often (particularly during the Progressive Era) the AMA has in fact been in the vanguard of attempts to reform health care organization and regulation, with enduring benefits to consumers as well as the physician profession. At any given juncture, AMA members are as often politically divided as unified over what public policies would in fact be best for physicians and the health care system as a whole. Yet, on the biggest issues, particularly the desirability of a nationalized health care system, AMA members are more unified and politically active than those of other interest groups, which accounts for the organization's relative political success. However, Burrow is rather pessimistic about the future ability of the AMA to respond adequately to the health care agenda he sees developing in the Sixties.

In a remarkably prophetic final chapter ("Survey of a Decade"), he commends the organization for its concerns regarding economic freedom and professional autonomy, but fears that it will be politically overwhelmed due to its inability to see how rapidly the nation's health care needs are changing. For an indeterminate future, the Association has set before itself enormous tasks. It seeks not only to provide the nation with adequate health care, but through methods that have been forcefully challenged in the United States and largely discarded abroad (p. 396). Any efforts to change this, he adds, will be hampered by an excessively decentralized organizational structure. Yet the AMA must change, for its own good as well as that of the nation's health care system. The contemporary scholar of American health policy, with the advantage of hindsight, can appreciate the acuity of Burrow's analysis.

In the Sixties, AMA's political inflexibility did lead to major legislative defeats over Medicare and Medicaid. Yet the organization recovered, reorganized, became more politically flexible and has effectively continued its efforts to preserve a largely private sector-administered (if not financed) health care system. With his superb understanding of the essential duality of AMA political impulses - part reformism, part reaction, with alternating periods of political inflexibility and pragmatism—James Burrow would certainly be able to understand what has happened to the publication of this well-crafted history.

14. Coulter, Harris L. *Divided Legacy: Volume III—Science and Ethics in American Medicine*: 1800 - 1914. Washington, DC: Wehawken Book Company, 1973.

This work is part of a larger series by the author that is intended to constitute a general history of medical thought. The book is organized into eight parts (covering over five hundred pages). Its primary topic is the clash between "allopathic" and "homeopathic" medicine. The author is generally sympathetic to the homeopaths, and concludes that the allopathic triumph in the 19th and early 20th Centuries is destined to be temporary, since it has left us with a medicine that de-emphasizes humanity, and is overly reliant on pharmaceuticals and technology. The author examines the participation by the AMA in the allopath homeopath controversy throughout the book. The founders of the AMA--particularly Nathan Smith Davis--were bitterly opposed to homeopathy, feeling it to be illogical, unscientific, and pandering to public superstition. However, the basic reason for AMA hostility to the homeopaths was economic. There is substantial evidence that homeopaths were more affluent than allopaths (who made up most of the AMA's membership). The Association, concerned about low doctors' income, wanted to restrict competition and improve the economic well-being of allopaths. In addition, the fact that homeopathy appealed to women was irritating to the largely male ranks of the AMA.

Quoting extensively from newspaper and journal articles, the author describes the determined (and often unscrupulous) efforts of the AMA to standardize medical education, restrict advertising, ban consultations and work for governmental regulation in order to eradicate the homeopathic influence. When some AMA members in New York arranged a truce, the national Association responded by expelling the New York State Medical Society. The AMA simply could not tolerate any threatening diversity in medical practice--even if the vast majority of the American public wanted such diversity. The AMA's concern for public and medical education in effect became a desire for the inculcation of allopathic orthodoxy. According to Coulter, "by 1910 the American Medical Association had absolute control over the future of American medicine" (p. 419). The homeopaths (as one might expect from a movement that preached diversity in medical practice) were divided, relatively disorganized and on the decline. In alliance with the pharmaceutical industry, the AMA itself was wealthy and organizationally effective. With the advent of the Flexner Report and the reorganization of medical education along AMA lines, the homeopathic movement collapsed, though its ideas may return in the future.

15. Duffy, John. *The Healers.* New York, NY: McGraw-Hill Book Company, 1976.

Subtitled "The Rise of the Medical Establishment," this book is a general history of American medicine. It contains twenty-one chapters (342 text pages) that follow a straightforward chronology from "The Myth of Indian Medicine" and "Health Conditions in the New World" to "Medicine Today." The author, Priscilla Alden Burke, Professor of History at the University of Maryland, has written extensively on U.S. medical history.

The book provides a basic outline of the impact of the American Medical Association on the nation's health care system. The initial motivations of the AMA are presented--improving the economic well-being of physicians, encouraging educational reform, and destroying the "sects" that the more orthodox members of the Association felt were undermining the profession. Until 1904, however, when it established an ongoing committee on education, its impact in that area was not great. In 1907 this committee requested the Carnegie Foundation to do its own research on medical schools. This led to Abraham Flexner's famous study. With respect to the ensuing educational reforms, the author asserts that "while Flexner could take justifiable pride in these changes, much of the credit belongs to the AMA Council on Medical Education, which, through its annual rating system, exerted continuous pressure to raise educational standards" (p. 265).

The AMA was not reform-minded in all areas, however. The Association began considering the issue of admitting female doctors to its ranks in 1868, but did not finally do so until 1915. Black physicians were even more firmly rejected by the AMA.

As a consequence, black local medical societies expanded, and the National Medical Association was established in 1895. AMA disapproval of contract medicine also slowed the growth of group practices until recent years.

Besides education, the AMA promoted reform efforts in the area of drug regulation and physician licensing. In 1906, it supported the successful push to enact the Pure Food and Drug Act. "Assisted by state and federal drug officials, the AMA continued to struggle to expose quackery and to strengthen the drug laws" (p. 296) in ensuing years. The Association worked for the passage of the Food, Drug and Cosmetic Act of 1938. To lessen the impact of state-by-state variation in medical groups, the AMA supported the establishment of the National Board of Medical Examiners in 1915.

Dr. Duffy provides a short history of the AMA in "Medical Licensure, Fees, and Societies" (Chapter 19) that stresses the progressive accomplishments of the organization. In the following chapter ("The Public's Health"), however, he argues that the AMA has lost credibility by its consistent opposition to most 20th Century social legislation in health care. Further obstructionism may be counterproductive: "In a democracy there are certain social and political realities; by facing up to them, physicians may well be able to write safeguards into new legislation, whereas blind opposition may bring on precisely what they most fear" (p. 314).

16. Fishbein, Morris. *A History of the American Medical Association 1847 to 1947*. Philadelphia, PA: W. B. Saunders Company, 1947.

This sprawling (over twelve hundred pages) volume contains the AMA's official history during the first hundred years of its existence, authored by a former editor of the Journal of the American Medical Association, Morris Fishbein. Despite its title, however, it contains the work of many other authors on a number of related topics, including AMA Presidents' biographies, descriptions of the various councils and bureaus of the Association, outlines of the AMA's publications and a number of historical appendices. Though it was published forty-five years ago, it is still an indispensable work for anyone wishing to understand the Association's own perceptions of its past and present development and professional mission.

The book begins with a short account (authored by Nathan Smith Davis III) of the professional development of Nathan Smith Davis, the founder of the American Medical Association. After a modest upbringing in Chenango County, New York, Smith eventually wound up receiving his physician training at the Medical College of Western New York. He joined the Broome County Medical Society in 1837, and became a delegate of the New York State Medical Society in 1844. Dissatisfied with professional standards, and frustrated by the inability of any one state society to materially change matters, he chaired a committee which called the 1847 meeting that established the AMA. He would eventually become the sixteenth and seventeenth Presidents of the organization--the only person to ever serve more than one term in that position. He would also write the first history of the AMA (published in 1855), and, in the words of the author, serve as "an 'untiring, irrepressible, uncompromising and incorruptible' leader" (p. 8).

The next five hundred pages of the text are taken up by Fishbein's "History," divided into 29 parts. Within each of the parts, significant AMA events between 1847 and 1947 are covered in strict chronology, set off by headings representing each year (with a few exceptions; 1861 and 1862, for example, are completely omitted, since there were no National Conventions during those years). Within each year, subheadings deal with individual items of concern (medical findings, new publications, committee deliberations, financial and recruitment matters, major items for debate at the National Convention and so forth). This makes the narrative choppier than it might have been with a more thematic organization. Some of the years are covered in one or two paragraphs, while others are given much greater treatment. In many years, the primary event covered is the AMA National Convention. The activities of the various journals and committees receive somewhat less attention, while state and local Association activities are brought up very infrequently. As one might expect in an official chronicle, the account provided, as well as the language, are decidedly positive toward the Association's establishment and growth. The idealistic motives of the AMA's "founding fathers" - an end to medical quackery, the firm linkage of medicine to science, and establishment of an effective code of ethics - are described; much less is mentioned about any possible aspirations to increase professional income and prestige. The wealth of detail, however (much of it taken from primary source material such as AMA Convention resolutions and debate), is unsurpassed.

To make Association actions more understandable, Fishbein occasionally links them to brief descriptions of health conditions in the larger society, and developments in medical technique and technology. The primary focus is nevertheless internal, with particular attention being paid to the happenings at annual conventions and the work of the various Association committees.

The rise of the Journal of the American Medical Association is extensively covered from every angle, including editorial and advertising policies and coverage of contemporary issues including the narrowly clinical (the dynamics of diphtheria and poliomyelitis); governmental/regulatory (the passage of pure food and drug legislation); and the merely quaint (the relationship between tightly-laced women's garments and gallstones).

Though Fishbein does not provide an extensive amount of personal analysis or commentary, the patient reader can gain a sense, year by year, of the gradual organizational expansion and elaboration of the Association and its increasing concern with public policy issues that impact upon the practice of medicine. Despite the Association's concern for physician independence, as time passes it becomes obvious that its goals of clinical professionalism and scientific medicine can only be achieved with the assistance of an actively regulatory government--first at the state levels, then in Washington. The largely successful efforts of the AMA to reach its ends through the advocacy of government action, are fully described (though, once again, in a disjointed, year-by-year, fashion). Of necessity, then, the latter parts of the history devote increasing attention to social and political concerns.

By 1905, the Association had established a Bureau of Medical Legislation and was vigorously engaged in public debates over "patent" medicines, "cults," public health, medical education, physician advertising and the proposed national prohibition of alcohol. After World War I, however, the issue of medical insurance, particularly proposals for government to provide it to all citizens ("socialized medicine," in Fishbein's terms), looms larger and larger. Fishbein's history records the vehement opposition of the Association to health insurance in resolution after resolution emanating from the National Conventions and the House of Delegates.

The history abruptly ends with the AMA's indictment and trial, on combination and conspiracy in restraint of trade charges (United States of America vs. the American Medical Association et al.) by a federal government that was ironically, to some extent, brought into medical matters by the AMA itself. The author was himself a principal figure in the trial, and there are extensive quotations provided from the testimony, as well as editorial cartoons from various newspapers providing commentary. On April 14, 1941, the trial ended with mixed results: all individual defendants were acquitted, but the AMA itself, and the District of Columbia Medical Society, were found guilty (though fined only $4000).

The next two sections of the text profile the nine recipients of the Distinguished Service Medal, and the 101 Presidents of the Association. The latter biographies are authored by Walter L. Bierring (who was himself the 87th AMA President), include a photograph of each president and average two to three pages in length. In addition to Association activities, they usually provide information on the educational background and professional accomplishments of each subject. Though each is brief, the profiles total almost three hundred pages of text.

The final two sections of the book have numerous authors, and provide descriptions of the then-existing twenty-one Councils and Bureaus of the Association, and the thirteen Association publications (though, oddly enough, not including the Journal itself). The sections on the Councils and Bureaus are more substantial than the previous biographies, ranging from five pages on the Bureau of Investigations to 36 pages on the Council on Medical Education and Hospitals. Both they and the journal accounts provide short developmental histories, including founding individuals (as with the above-mentioned biographies, often with photographs).

There are several appendices at the conclusion of the book. One lists the location of each yearly National Convention, the President of that convention, and the state he represented. Others list the membership of the Board of Trustees, the Judicial Council, and the Council on Medical Education and Hospitals. The attendance at each National Convention is also listed, as are important dates in the history of the Council on Medical Education and Hospitals. Those looking for a coherent vision of the historical purpose and objectives of the American Medical Association, and a detailed analysis of its actions, will have to supplement this with other works. But as a source of data on historical events, and the people who created the AMA and led it to preeminence the American health care system, this book has no equal. Any serious scholar of U.S. medical history must consider it required reading.

17. Haller, John S. Jr. *American Medicine in Transition 1840 - 1910*. Urbana, IL: University of Illinois Press, 1981.

The author is a Professor and Associate Vice President for Academic Affairs, as well as Dean of Graduate Studies, at California State University - Long Beach. His book examines the evolution of "Victorian medicine" in the U.S. between 1840 and 1910 (the year the Flexner Report was issued). In 323 text pages and nine chapters, the work covers both clinical and social issues in this development. There is also an extensive Notes section at the end.

According to Dr. Haller, "unlike European medical organizations which were national in authority and aristocratic in design, the American Medical Association evolved through a process that was democratic in design, national in authority and elitist in practice - much in keeping with many other developmental aspects of American society" (p. 212). The establishment of the AMA was primarily due to physicians' concerns with declining economic and social status. Above all, the Association saw reform in medical education as the key to reversing these adverse trends. Political activity was also necessary, so the AMA established a National Committee on Medical Legislation, a Legislative Council and a National Auxiliary Congressional and Legislative Committee. Contacts with state legislatures and the U.S. Congress steadily increased. The AMA proposed a clinical base for teaching, formalized cooperative efforts between hospitals and medical schools, stricter examination and licensing standards and an end to "sectarian" medical doctrines. On all of these proposals, however, the Association was effectively opposed by many medical schools. In response, the AMA excluded representatives of proprietary medical schools from its national meeting in 1874.

The AMA was also distracted from its reform efforts by constant factional conflict within the organization, particularly over its Code of Ethics, and frequent crusades against homeopaths. Dr. Haller terms the

AMA attacks upon sectarians "efforts to restrict freedom of the marketplace and the independence of sectarian believers" (p. 258).

The turning point for AMA efforts to influence medical education came with the Association's reorganization in 1904. In that year, the Association permanently established its Council on Medical Education, and undertook a deliberate effort "to expose and destroy the multitude of inferior medical schools by publishing the poor showing their graduates made on state medical exams" (p. 225). Between 1906 and 1910, the AMA's activities contributed to the closing of 29 schools. By 1908, the AMA was insisting upon inspection of all medical schools. To bolster its efforts, the Council on Medical Education "urged the selection of an impartial outsider to conduct a study of medical education" (p. 225). This led to the Flexner Report. Dr. Haller summarizes by classifying the AMA as a reforming, change-oriented institution much like the modern American corporation. "Like Rockefeller and Carnegie, the early history of the AMA had virtues which were largely ignored, let alone understood" (p. 233).

18. King, Lester S. *American Medicine Comes of Age: 1840-1920.* Chicago, IL: American Medical Association, 1984.

This is a short compilation of twenty-four essays that originally ran monthly from July 1982 to June 1984 in the *Journal of the American Medical Association* as "Medicine in the U.S.A.: Historical Vignettes". Designed to commemorate the 100th birthday of *JAMA*, the volume's essays deal with a variety of social, economic, political and legal issues that confronted medicine between 1840 and 1920. The author, Lester King, is a physician who has carried out medical history research and instruction at the Morris Fishbein Center at the University of Chicago, and is also a former editor of *JAMA*'s book review column.

The essays average five pages in length, and are arranged in chronological order. They begin by chronicling the British influence on early American medicine; move through developments in medical education and ethics, and the growing scientific content of medicine; and conclude with the impact of a modernizing America on a rapidly specializing physician profession. The most important milestones of this history, including the founding of the American Medical Association and *JAMA*, and the Flexner Report, are outlined. Dr. King also provides bibliographic notes with each essay for those readers who might wish to further explore a given topic. Dr. King writes well and concisely. He does not have any overarching theme or message of his own to propound, but nevertheless ties the essays together so that they read more like a single work of history than a collection of essays on a wide variety of topics. On the more technical subjects ("Germ Theory and its Influence," or "Medicine Seeks to be Scientific," for example), the description is adequately detailed, but written so that non-specialists can readily grasp the major points. Major contending viewpoints on controversial political and ethical issues ("The AMA Gets a New Code of Ethics" and "Medical Education: Elitism and Reform") are objectively presented and explained.

King also has a sharp eye for the connections between modern physician development and the socioeconomic and technological evolution of the larger society. This leads, among other things, to an unusual and informative essay relating turn-of-the-century medical practice to the newest mode of transportation ("The Automobile Makes an Impact"). Most importantly, Dr. King, like any good historian, realizes that historical accounts require analysis as well as description.

The final (and most thought-provoking) essay in the series, "The Continuity of History," provides the reader with his thoughts on the intricacies of attempting to develop a coherent picture of the past based upon often scattered and disputed fragments of old information. Using Robert Koch's discovery of the bacillus responsible for tuberculosis as his primary example, King shows how any understanding of the importance of this nineteenth century event requires a broad understanding of numerous contemporary concepts and issues in a variety of social, scientific and professional areas. Despite the practical difficulties, Dr. King sees no alternative to a history based upon the important connections between a wide range of natural and social factors. "The interrelation of events is, I believe, an important message of history. Perhaps the study of medical history will induce sympathy for this network approach with its concepts of interpenetration and continuity. These concepts, I suggest, are really the foundation of all of medicine, and not merely of its history" (p. 115).

19. Konold, Donald E. *A History of American Medical Ethics 1847 - 1912.* Madison, WI: State Historical Society of Wisconsin, 1962.

This short (75 text pages) work is a doctoral dissertation for the Department of History at the University of Missouri. In it, the author provides an overview of the development of medical ethics in the U.S. divided into six topical chapters: "The Establishment of Ethical Control," "The Regulation of Quackery," "The Relation of Research to Medical Ethics," "The Relations of Physicians to Laymen," "The Ethics of Money" and "The Course of Ethical Regulation".

As Dr. Konold points out, the members of the American Medical Association expressed concern about the state of medical ethics at the second convention of the organization in 1847. The Association formally adopted a "Code of Ethics," which in turn was largely derived from a code drafted by an English physician, Thomas Percival, in 1796. "The Association's Code dealt with the relationships of physicians to one another, to their patients and to the public, and paid less attention to other matters" (p. 10). It would not be significantly modified until 1903.

During the latter half of the 1800's, actual adherence to the Code was largely voluntary. The apprentice system of education led to wide variation in levels of professional competence. The AMA preached against commercialism and "quackery" in medicine, but was generally unsuccessful in its efforts to convince states to pass laws banning such practices until the turn of the century. However, the AMA was more successful in encouraging physicians to avoid consultations with doctors who engaged in "irregular practices". Efforts to oppose unethical medical practices blended into the larger AMA opposition to medical "sects". Regarding "the ethics of money," the AMA generally opposed contract practices, arguing that they led to undercharging.

In 1903, the AMA relegated its Code to advisory status, turning its attention to the promotion of scientific medicine. It did, however, adopt the Principles of Medical Ethics in 1912. This new resolution was primarily concerned with the right of the AMA to discipline wayward members if necessary. In practice, the responsibility for ethical monitoring devolved to the state and local medical societies. The area of public health was an exception to this. AMA support for the public health movement included ethically-oriented injunctions on the need for physicians to report infectious diseases, and general interest in "such varied matters as school hygiene, vaccination, abortion, control of venereal disease and prostitution, alcoholism and--by the end of the century--the campaign against tuberculosis" (p. 53). In 1910, the Association established a Council on Health and Public Instruction, which prepared written educational materials for public release and provided a Speaker's Bureau.

From 1910 until 1957, the AMA focused on a relatively small number of ethical issues. The Association's concern over the use of physicians as expert witnesses in court hearings led to proposals (largely unheeded by state legislatures, and abandoned by the AMA by 1914) that courts appoint other doctors to serve as independent arbiters, with binding legal powers, on such testimony. The practice of fee-splitting met with vigorous AMA condemnation. The Association constantly attacked any form of advertising as potentially unethical. And, above all, compulsory health insurance (especially if any government was involved) was rejected.

In Chapter 6 ("The Course of Ethical Regulation"), Dr. Konold concludes that amendments to the Principles of Medical Ethics since

1912 have largely involved efforts to restrict commercial practices and preserve physicians' (and the AMA's) economic and clinical prerogatives. Practical enforcement of other ethical concerns has been irregular at best. "Though medical leaders repeatedly dedicated their profession to the cause of human welfare, they invariably confounded their idealism by asserting the dubious proposition that the profession could best serve society by serving itself" (p. 75).

20. Numbers, Ronald L., Editor. *The Education of American Physicians*. Berkeley, CA: University of California Press, 1980.

This is a book of historical essays, written by a variety of historians and clinicians, and edited by the Chairman of the Department of the History of Medicine at the University of Wisconsin -Madison. The introduction and thirteen essays cover approximately three hundred pages, and range from preclinical and clinical ("Anatomy" and "Surgery") to social scientific ("Medical Ethics and Jurisprudence," "Medical History") subjects. Several of the authors deal with the historical impact of the American Medical Association on medical education.

In "American Medical Education," Martin Kaufman briefly recounts the concerns about low quality education that lay behind the establishment of the AMA, and the efforts of the Chicago Medical College (with Nathan Smith Davis, a founder of the AMA, as an influential faculty member) to provide a high quality medical education. He also discusses how the AMA worked for educational reform through the Association of American Medical Colleges (established in 1890) and its Council on Medical Education (formed in 1893).

John Harley Warner ("Physiology"), David L. Cowen ("Materia Medica and Pharmacology"), Russell C. Maulitz ("Pathology"), Edward C. Atwater ("Internal Medicine") and Jeanne L. Brand ("Neurology and Psychiatry") all list the efforts the AMA made to upgrade relevant curricular materials and experiences. In 1852, the AMA recommended that each medical school have sixteen weeks of instruction in Materia Medica, while an Association report elaborated upon weaknesses in physiology instruction in 1907.

The 1909 AMA model curriculum emphasized the need for high quality laboratory instruction and equipment in pathology (though there was also evidence of a growing split between pathology and bacteriology). Internal medicine was an enduring preoccupation for the AMA, with efforts to promote the greater use of hospitals (and less reliance upon college clinics for practical experience). And by 1940 the AMA Section on Nervous and Mental Disease had endorsed the establishment of a neuropsychiatric institute that would eventually become NIMH. With respect to "Public Health and Preventive Medicine," Judith Walzer Leavitt outlines the strong AMA interest in the area since its inception. Its advocacy increased after the Civil War, and hygiene and medical police were included in the proposed four-year curriculum that the AMA issued in 1871. The AMA, allied with the Committee on the Teaching of Hygiene of the APHA and the AAMC, "supported advanced training for specialists in public health in addition to basic training in hygiene for all medical students" (p. 257).

The topics of "Medical Ethics and Jurisprudence"(Chester R. Burns) were initially tied in with the long-lasting conflict within the AMA over codes of medical ethics. Legal and ethical topics were covered in lectures, but formal courses in either area were not common until the 1930s. In 1927, the AMA's Council on Medical Education called for the development of a course entitled "social relations of the physician," which would contain legal and ethical material. The AMA has continued to support instruction in these areas.

21. Rosenberg, Charles E., Editor. *Healing and History: Essays for George Rosen.* Kent, England: Wm. Davidson & Sons, Ltd., 1979.

A collection of essays on various aspects of medical history, this work is dedicated to the late George Rosen, the prominent medical historian. Its sixteen essays cover approximately 250 pages, and their topics range from "Medical Ethics and Honoraria in Late Antiquity" to "The American Journal of Public Health, 1957-1973."

In "C.E.A. Winslow: His Era and His Contribution to Medical Care," Arthur J. Viseltear of Yale University looks at Winslow's work as vice chairman for the Committee on the Cost of Medical Care between 1927 and 1932. The objective of the committee was to develop a reorganization plan for American health care. Initially, Winslow optimistically hoped for the cooperation and support of the American Medical Association in the committee's efforts. Olin West, the Executive Secretary of the AMA, was in face a member of the committee. The committee's report attempted to provide a compromise between the attitudes and needs of physicians and medical reformers. "But despite [Winslow's] appeals...the AMA and its spokesmen remained adamantly opposed to change" (p. 219). The report received a great deal of criticism from the AMA, and its proposals were never adopted.

(B) Articles

22. Baker, Samuel L. "A Strange Case: The Physician Licensure Campaign in Massachusetts in 1880." *Journal of the History of Medicine and Allied Sciences* 40(3) (July, 1985): 206-208.

Baker's case study is concerned with physician licensure laws and State laws that restrict those who wish to professionally practice medicine. He addresses the advocacy of such licensure by medical societies in existence in the 1800's. In this historical view of licensure in Massachusetts, the American Social Science Association was the facilitator of licensure legislation for the state. The AMA adamantly opposed the membership of homeopaths and eclectic, and those that advocated their licensure as professional physicians.

23. Berlant, Jeffrey L. "Medical Ethics and Professional Monopoly." *The Annals of the American Academy of Internal Medicine* 437 (1978): 49-61.

The author, as a Diplomat of the American Board of Internal Medicine, discusses how the evolution of medical ethics is related to socio-economic factors that changed over the years. Berlant first reviews the ethics developed by Thomas Percival in England and contrasts those by John Gregory in Scotland.

The author then shows how the AMA began by adopting the ethics of Percival but then changed them in response to occurrences such as passage of the Sherman Anti-Trust Act of 1898. Berlant maintains that much of the AMA's ethics promoted monopolistic practices such as fee fixing, the necessity of physicians being their own evaluators of competence, and professional hegemony in all new medical care arrangements such as prepaid plans or federally sponsored health services.

24. King, Lester S. "The Painfully Slow Progress in Medical Education." *Journal of the American Medical Association* 249(2) (January 14, 1983): 94-96.

This historical vignette by Dr. King accounts a half century of slow progress towards improving medical education in the U.S. The author points out that the AMA, in its very first year of 1847, voiced the common criticism of existing medical education. There was widespread agreement that preliminary educational requirements should be bolstered. Second, that medical schools should offer longer periods of instruction (e.g., six vs. four months). Third, the course itself should be graded, disciplines expanded and more clinical teaching included. Would-be reformers criticized the serious glut in poorly prepared doctors, produced by proprietary schools where instructors' income depended upon the number of students enrolled. These reformers therefore advocated separate examiners for medical school graduation and readiness to actually practice medicine.

Dr. King includes historical background on debated topics such as the value of lectures, and whether a two-tiered approach should be used. One to educate and prepare students for practice and a second tier of students who would learn more and perform research to advance scientific medical knowledge.

25. King, Lester S. "The Founding of the American Medical Association." *Journal of the American Medical Association* 248(14) (October 8, 1982): 1749-1752.

King's historical vignette accounts the background events and conditions leading up to the 1847 founding of the AMA. The author reviews the earlier work by state medical societies and their concern for quality education, medical ethics, scientific practice and meaningful state licensing of physicians. Dr. King reviews actions of the New York state Medical Society and their response to the State's 1844 revocation of special privileges of the regular medical profession. This is an excellent summary of why and how a guild organized and furthered its professional interests by regulating its profession through ethics, educational standards, gatekeeping, and related actions.

26. King, Lester S. "The Founding of *JAMA*, 1883." *Journal of the American Medical Association* 250(2) (August 1983): 177-180.

Dr. King provides another excellent article in his historical vignette series with this one on the Journal of the American Medical Association (*JAMA*). The author documents the several motives for creating *JAMA*, which include timely distribution of scientific papers, strengthening of AMA membership and providing a source of revenues through selling advertisements in the Journal. Dr. King accounts how AMA President Lewis A. Sayre advocated using the British Medical Association's Journal as a model. The British had quickly quadrupled their association's membership by automatically making all subscribers members of their Association. After several years of AMA Committee study, *JAMA* was finally given approval and first published July 14, 1883 with an initial circulation of 31,800. By 1898, *JAMA* circulation was 11,270, while AMA membership was only 8,000. Although it initially was not the remarkable success of its British counterpart, the *JAMA* did succeed in fulfilling all of its objectives and has become a quality journal honored worldwide by the medical profession.

27. King, Lester S. "The AMA Gets a New Code of Ethics." *Journal of the American Medical Association* 249(10) (March 11, 1983): 1335-1342.

The author provides historical background of AMA's revised Code of Ethics of 1903. This revision was in heated debate for over 20 years. The central issue was whether the code would continue to prohibit regular scientific physicians from consulting with homeopaths and other "sects." While homeopaths now had their own medical schools and had come a long way in adopting "scientific methods," they remained a serious irritant to the "regulars" for continuing to declare themselves a separate sect and criticizing the "regulars." The issue led to fragmentation of State Medical Societies in New York and constant debate within AMA in the 1880's and 90's. Finally, a new AMA code of ethics was adopted in 1903, which no longer prohibited consultation with homeopaths or other sects; the code did, however, state it was incompatible for honorable physicians to designate their practice based on exclusive dogma.

28. Nickens, Herbert W. "A Case of Professional Exclusion in 1870 - the Formation of the First Black Medical Society." *Journal of the American Medical Association* 253(17) (May 3, 1985): 2549 -2552.

Dr. Nickens' article looks at organized medicine in the 1860's and 1870's, and its successful attempt to exclude black physicians from joining the local medical society in Washington, D.C. As a result of this resistance to accept minorities, the first black medical society was formed as the local branch of the National Medical Society. Simultaneously, the AMA voted in 1871 to continue excluding delegates from Colleges that included women. Nickens concludes that, in 1985, medicine is taking on a more corporate face, patients are being viewed as consumers and may increasingly receive health care based on their ability to pay; and that, says the author, means blacks may face a further deterioration in their relative health status.

29. Centennial Issue, *Journal of the American Medical Association* 250(2) (July 8, 1983).

This 1983 Centennial Issue is a reprint of the first *JAMA* issue originally printed July 14, 1883. For those without access to the first and rare copy of *JAMA*, this Centennial Issue is a highly welcome edition. The reader can better appreciate the magnitude and financial importance of *JAMA* advertising to AMA funding. In addition, this issue includes minutes of the AMA's annual convention of 1883, AMA President Atlee's annual address, scientific and medical articles, editorials, medical society items and miscellany. The issue provides the reader with a better understanding of the concerns of organized medicine in 1883, as well as the "advancements" or medical progress of interest in that era.

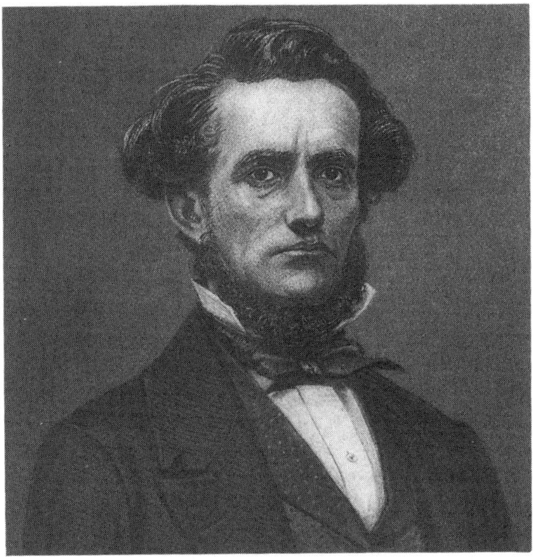

Source: Nathan Smith Davis, M.D., *History of the American Medical Association from Its Organization up to January, 1855.* Philadelphia: Lippincott, Grambo, & Co., 1855.

Dr. Nathan Smith Davis founded the American Medical Association in 1847.

Davis was born January 9, 1817 in a log cabin near Green, New York. He graduated in 1837 from the College of Physicians and Surgeons of Western New York in Fairfield, New York. In July of 1837, Davis started his medical practice in Binghamton, New York.

In 1838, Dr. Davis married Anna-Maria Parker. Davis was a leader in founding the AMA in 1846 and 1847. In 1849, he accepted the Chair of Physiology and Pathology at Rush Medical College in Chicago. By 1850, Dr. Davis was active in helping organize state and local medical societies and starting the Illinois General Hospital of the Great Lakes.

In 1854, Dr. Davis became Vice President of the AMA. In 1855, he published the association's first history. Davis went on to help start the medical department of Lind University--later renamed the Northwestern University Medical School.

From 1864 to 1866, Dr. Davis served as AMA President. In 1868, he introduced a resolution to begin the AMA Library. Dr. Davis became the first editor of the Journal of the AMA in 1882.After serving the AMA for over 40 years, Dr. Davis died in 1904.

4

THE ASSOCIATION DEVELOPS (1901 - PRESENT)

The readings in this section outline the development of the American Medical Association, to the peak of power and then relative decline, during this century. The AMA grew rapidly in membership and political influence in the first decade of the 1900s. In alliance with "reform" elements within medical schools and state legislatures, and more generally as part of the Progressive political movement, the AMA and its Council on Medical Education were able to bring about the increased regulation (generally in the direction of more rigorous standards) of medical school education and clinical practice in many states between 1900 and 1910. Most importantly, in the latter part of the decade, AMA leaders were instrumental in the establishment of Abraham Flexner's study of U.S. medical education (albeit funded by the Carnegie Foundation). Once issued, the Flexner Report brought about the final triumph of the reformers, and--not coincidentally--the rise of the AMA to the status of semi-official national arbiter of medical education and practice standards. By the 1920's, the AMA-led reform coalition reigned supreme over American medical practice.

The success of the AMA, however, ironically brought about an evolution in the structure of U.S. health care that was to gradually reduce the organization's strength in the decades to come. "Scientific medicine" led to physician specialization, and medical specialists often became more interested in their subfield than the physician profession as a whole. The AMA therefore lost a critical degree of support among the doctors it professed to recognize. The expansion of effective medical knowledge and technology that also came from "scientific medicine" led to increased levels of public demand for health services, and gradually increasing costs for those services. The movement for health insurance, which had begun during the Progressive Era but stalled during the 1920's period of "normalcy", was revived and would build momentum throughout the middle decades of the century.

Now an increasingly wealthy part of the medical Establishment, many physicians, led by the AMA, moved to the right politically. The Association was firmly dominated by solo fee-for-service practitioners whose leaders (most notably, Morris Fishbein, editor of JAMA) opposed almost all governmental health programs as "socialism". But the Great Depression during the Thirties, and the Second World War in the 1940s, irrevocably committed the Federal Government to domestic activism and intervention. And the growing need for revenues to fuel "modern medicine" led even the AMA to accept such Federal initiatives as the Hill-Burton Hospital Construction Act of 1946. The growing public clamor for more physicians (as well as revenue shortfalls) gradually overcame AMA and medical school resistance to public funding, so Federal subsidies also began to flow into medical education through such avenues as the Health Professions Education Assistance Act of 1963.

When rising social concerns about health care for the poor and elderly were heard by politicians in the Kennedy and Johnson Administrations, AMA resistance to any significant changes within the structure of U.S. medical services was clearly out of step with majority sentiments. In 1965, Medicare and Medicaid, national health insurance programs for the poor and elderly, were enacted by Congress. The common prediction was that a comprehensive, governmentally-managed national health program would follow them into law within ten years.

However, as in the Progressive Era, public confidence in governmental activism waned as the Johnson Administration saw failure after failure in its Great Society and Vietnam War efforts. The AMA was politically flexible and intelligent enough to accept that the national government was now a permanent player in the health field. The Association turned its attention toward ensuring that governmental efforts would enhance the prosperity and prerogatives of physicians, and was largely successful. Doctors received more and more income from governmental sources, yet their operational activities were not significantly controlled. American health care costs began to rise rapidly, as cost containment replaced access as the chief health policy concern. Voluntary cost control efforts promoted by the Nixon and Ford Administrations failed.

The AMA, in alliance with hospital interests, fought and restrained the Carter Administration's hospital cost control proposals. But when the Reagan Administration entered office and embraced the doctrines of health care competition and cost containment, the AMA faced a fundamental challenge to the physician-dominated, fee-for-service medical system that had been the greatest legacy of AMA activity in the twentieth century. With the rise of a payor-dominated market system, increased corporate involvement in health care management, and major efforts to limit hospital (prospective payment systems) and physician (Resource Based Relative Value Systems) charges, it was clear that the unique role that physicians and the AMA had fulfilled within the American health care system since the Flexner Report was gone forever. As it did at the end of the previous century, the Association and its members would face a new, and uncertain, future.

(A) Books

30. Anderson, Odin W. *The Uneasy Equilibrium.* New Haven, CT: College & University Press, 1968.

As the subtitle of this book ("Private and Public Financing of Health Services in the United States, 1875-1965") indicates, Dr. Anderson focuses on money in health care--where it has come from, and what it has been spent on. Odin Anderson is a Professor and member of the Center for Health Administration Studies at the University of Chicago. His book is just over two hundred pages in length, and covers its subject in five parts: "The Development of the Health Services 1875-1915", "The Economic Problems of Patients 1915-1935", "Adoption of the Principles of Health Insurance 1933-1952", "Problems and Issues Within the Consensus 1948-1965", and "Continuing Challenge and Response".

Dr. Anderson examines the attitudes of the American Medical Association regarding financing policy, and its resulting political activity, in a number of places in his narrative. He notes that in 1915, JAMA editorials forwarded arguments in favor of health insurance, and called upon physicians to work with state legislators to develop acceptable programs. The AMA formed a Committee on Social Insurance, which "was motivated by a great deal of legitimate professional self-interest" (p. 71).

AMA national activity on the health insurance question diminished during World War I, but state societies became heavily involved in deliberations within their respective legislatures. By 1919, however, physician opinion at the state level had turned strongly against all forms of health insurance. At the 1920 annual convention, the AMA House of Delegates passed a resolution that declared "its opposition to the institution of any plan embodying the system of compulsory contribution insurance . . . provided, controlled, or regulated by any state or the Federal Government" (p. 74). Subsequent AMA resolutions elaborated upon organizational opposition to "state medicine", holding that any governmental intervention into health services (with the sole and narrowly defined exception of public health functions) was illegitimate. The Association also opposed the findings of the Committee on the Cost of Health Care, released in 1932, comparing government health insurance to socialism and Communism.

Dr. Anderson outlines subsequent AMA successes in keeping health insurance schemes out of the 1935 Social Security Act, and preventing subsequent Congressional proposals from enaction. The Association engaged in extensive negotiation with Congress in the development of "eldercare" legislation in the early Sixties, attempting to simultaneously support the general concept but ensure policy specifics that conformed to AMA notions of physician prerogatives and autonomy. This time, however, its activities were unsuccessful, and Medicare was passed over AMA opposition. Anderson notes that "the AMA suffered a defeat in the passage of Medicare, and although its opposition to government health insurance will doubtlessly continue, the Association will not be as strong a rallying point for those who are likely to oppose health care legislation at the national level in the future" (p. 198). The author concludes by expressing his optimism regarding a future moderation toward the insurance issue by all major policy participants.

31. Bowers, John S. *An Introduction to American Medicine--1975*. Washington, DC: U.S. Government Printing Office, 1977.

This is a publication of the U.S. Department of Health, Education and Welfare, Public Health Service and the National Institutes of Health. The author is a former Dean and Professor of both the University of Utah and University of Wisconsin medical schools, and is currently head of the Josiah Macy, Jr. Foundation. Containing 208 text pages, the monograph is divided into five chapters, each focusing on one particular aspect of U.S. health care: "The Patient", "The Physician", "Education and Research", "Hospitals", and "Medical Care".

According to Dr. Bowers in "Physicians", the American Medical Association has historically been the "mother" of U.S. doctors. For a long time, its various sections and journals met the needs (and earned the loyalty) of both specialists and general practitioners. However, at some time in recent history, "the AMA began to fall from 'divine' grace" (p. 33). Specialists (growing in number due to the rapid advances in physician practice) turned to their particular societies to meet their needs. Even the general practitioners have found another organization (the American Academy of Family Physicians) to work within. The author argues that some of the AMA's membership loss is due to its increasing focus on political and economic issues, and its general opposition to many medical innovations (such as group practice and prepaid health care) that younger physicians support. Despite efforts by the AMA to change in response to these developments, Dr. Bowers concludes that the organization will never regain the preeminence that it once had.

The author describes a number of the AMA's historical activities and policy positions in "Medical Care" (Chapter 5). The Association vigorously opposed the development of group practices, going to court against the Group Health Association in 1937 and the Group Health Cooperative of Puget Sound in 1946. The AMA also contended that prepaid group practices violated the principle of free choice of physician by patient, and also were unfairly competitive with fee-for-service practitioners. After a number of legal defeats, the AMA revised its policies to accept some forms of group practices, including PGPs.

National health insurance proposals met with particularly strong AMA opposition. Initially, the Association opposed any medical benefits under Social Security. Dr. Bowers also briefly describes the AMA efforts to derail the passage of Medicare legislation. After Medicare was enacted, the AMA continued to pay attention to its implementation, criticizing HEW efforts to limit allowable drug costs and defending doctors against the charges of widespread fraud under the program. More recently, the AMA has attempted to legally block the inception of the National Health Planning and Resources Development Act of 1974 (Public Law 93-641). "The AMA contends that the act is in direct violation of the Constitution, since it transfers to Federal control authority which has been constitutionally reserved for the States, thereby, the AMA claims, placing the control of health facilities and ultimately the control of the practice of medicine in the Federal bureaucracy" (p. 189).

32. Burrow, James G. *Organized Medicine in the Progressive Era.* Baltimore, MD: Johns Hopkins University Press, 1977.

This work grew out of Burrow's previous investigation of the historical development of the American Medical Association (*AMA: Voice of Organized Medicine*), and is both shorter (approximately 150 pages of text) and focused on one particular period in American history, the Progressive Era. During these first two decades of the Twentieth Century, social and professional reform movements transformed American physician education and practice into highly efficient and scientifically-based processes. They also facilitated the rise of monopoly-based physician power over the entire health care system. Burrow shows how these changes came about in a readable and well-organized volume. In doing so, he also continues to emphasize the complex and important point established in his earlier work: the essential duality of AMA principles and behavior. Both deeply idealistic and intensely self-interested, the Association and its members made enormous contributions to the quality and safety of American medicine even as they established systemwide controls that enhanced their own wealth and privileges.

The book contains ten chapters, and is divided into three parts. Part II, "Ferment and Reform," recounts how the physician reformers, eventually led by the AMA, achieved their aims. The AMA vigorously attacked the wide variety of "healing sects," such as Christian Science and osteopathy, for "unsound and dangerous practices" that should be prohibited. The AMA's Council on Medical Education pushed states and universities for educational reforms buttressed by more stringent legal requirements for licensure. The basic objective was usually to persuade governments to control the practice of health care, and to utilize only the standards and judgments of physicians in setting up such controls.

Despite their status as relative political amateurs, the AMA-led physician reformers were almost uniformly successful in getting their vision of health care administration enacted into law. In Part III ("Matters of Economics"), Burrow discusses how this vision led to unprecedented physician control over health care. Brushing past antitrust legislation, physicians emulated Big Business in establishing monopoly control (supported by law) over the provision of health services. As Burrow suggests in a short but effective summary, the Progressive Era ended with a growing and powerful AMA, and physicians firmly at the helm of the U.S. health care system. This set the stage for the controversies over the power and prerogatives of doctors that would arise in the latter half of the century.

33. Davis, Michael M. *America Organizes Medicine*. New York: Harper and Row, 1941.

This is a very thorough description of the many events and movements that have shaped organized medicine in American culture during the 20th century. The role of the AMA is discussed in descriptions that pertain to the influence of policy in maternal and child health care in which the AMA "bitterly opposed" providing federal grants to states in this area (i.e. opposition to the Sheppard-Towner Act of 1921). The role of the AMA in shaping standards for hospital "inspection" was also discussed. A very intriguing chapter of the book that inadvertently provides a historical perspective on how our definition of "quality" has changed is Chapter 13, titled "Yardsticks of Service". After stating that the President of the AMA, Nathan B. Van Etten, regarded the quality of care in America as the highest of any country, the author goes on to define quality as "competency of technical performance in any kind of service". This definition seems to have dominated the thinking in medical education and practice until very recently when a new quality paradigm (Continuous Quality Improvement) began to take hold.

34. Flexner, Abraham. *The Flexner Report on Medical Education in the United States and Canada, 1910.* New York, NY: the Carnegie Commission, 1910.

The most influential work on medical education in American history, this report by Abraham Flexner is more often cited than read by health services scholars and policymakers. Nevertheless, the reader, like the Carnegie Commission, will find a wealth of important and interesting information about past American medical educational patterns, a state-by-state rundown on medical school structures and functioning circa 1910, and an absorbing discussion on the "proper basis of medical education." In large part, the latter component outlines the current national design and curriculum for the education of physicians. The Flexner Report can thus be read both as history, and as a still-relevant health educational policy document.

Despite its breadth and depth of coverage, the Flexner Report is surprisingly concise--only slightly over three hundred pages. In an Introduction, Carnegie Foundation President Henry S. Pritchett summarizes the study's findings of excessive commercialism in medical education, a consequent production of poorly-trained doctors, and frequent failings with respect to technical facilities, curriculum and educational methods. He concludes that "in view of these facts, progress for the future would seem to require a very much smaller number of medical schools, better equipped and better conducted than our schools now as a rule are; and the needs of the public would equally require that we have fewer physicians graduated each year, but that they should be better educated and better trained" (p. xi).

The text of Flexner's report is divided into two parts. Part I, containing fourteen chapters, covers the history of American medical education, sets forth both the "proper" and "actual" bases for such education, and provides a detailed description of curricular, financial and governance matters. It also has separate chapters on "the medical education of women" and "the medical education of the Negro."

Part II provides a factual description and analysis of each medical school in 37 states (listed in alphabetical order), the District of Columbia, and Canada. In his history, Abraham Flexner begins around 1750. His major conclusion is that the first medical schools were in fact "soundly conceived as organically part of an institution of learning and intimately connected with a large public hospital. (But) the sound start of these early schools was not long maintained. Their scholarly ideals were soon compromised and then forgotten" (pp. 4-5). He sees the basic reasons for this deterioration stemming from a lack of centralized and professional direction, and a growing commercial exploitation that grew out of the ever-present need for operating funds. He contemptuously brushes aside justifications for the status quo, and declares that "in modern life the medical profession is an organ differentiated by society for its own highest purposes, not a business to be exploited by individuals according to their own fancy . . . the time is surely ripe for decisive action" (p. 19).

Flexner then sets forth "the proper basis for medical education". This involves at least two years of undergraduate college education, including adequate foundations in chemistry, biology, physics and laboratory techniques. Ideally, it should also entail enough instruction in unspecified social and cultural topics to make the prospective physician "an educated man" (p. 26). Flexner declares, however, that "the actual basis of medical education" is all too often held to be at the high school or equivalency level, or even lower in some states. Lax or nonexistent state regulation of medical school admissions aggravates the problem of student quality. As a result, the caliber of medical student bodies varies from adequate (in only a handful of cases) to abysmal. Flexner concludes that schools must sharply raise admission standards, and opposition to this on the grounds of inadequate physician supply or (more covertly) the survival of commercial schools must be overcome.

In the following four chapters, Flexner analyzes the curricular path to a medical degree, including laboratory studies, medical school training and hospital experience. He examines both historical and contemporary practices, and strongly advocates a scientific orientation for both medical students and faculty, particularly in the areas of anatomy, physiology, pharmacology, pathology and bacteriology. This scientific orientation in turn strengthens the case for strong linkages between medical schools and other science departments within a university setting. Unfortunately, as with admissions, Flexner concludes that most operating medical schools fall far short of these requirements.

In the third and fourth years of medical school, Flexner sees the need for students to combine their classroom knowledge with well-integrated clinical instruction. According to him, "the test of a good education in medicine is the thorough interpenetration of both standpoints in their product, the young graduate" (p. 92). This entails work in medicine, surgery, obstetrics, and various specialties. Flexner goes on to discuss a variety of issues related to the proper structure and techniques of clinical instruction. Some medical schools, such as those at Johns Hopkins University, the University of Michigan, and Jefferson Medical College, are singled out for praise of their curricula, facilities and operating procedures. Others are excoriated for numerous inadequacies, often in wickedly caustic and colorful language. "Many of the schools mention in the course of this recital are probably without redeeming features of any kind. Their general squalor consorts well with their clinical poverty. . . In wretched amphitheaters students wait in vain for 'professors', tardy or absent, amusing the interval with ribald jest and song" (p. 124).

The remaining topics in Part I are covered in similar fashion. Given the scientific foundations of medical education, the schools dominated by "The Medical Sects" (allopathy, osteopathy and homeopathy) must either meet the above-outlined standards, or be outlawed. Flexner very briefly discusses "The Medical Education of Women" and "the Negro", but only to emphasize that appropriate educational opportunities for these groups should exist, and should involve the same scientific principles as earlier outlined.

The chapter on "Financial Aspects" dwells at length on the necessary operational costs of medical education, including the relationships with a hospital to provide clinical opportunities. He summarizes the matter by stating that "it is now clear that medicine cannot be, and is not, properly taught on the basis of receipts" (p. 136). Other, more secure sources of revenue must be obtained. Flexner admits in "Reconstruction" that, along with quality requirements, reform will necessitate a sharp reduction in the number of existing medical schools. Along with this, "The State Boards" must be strengthened, given their often scandalously weak current status. Their powers to mandate sound medical schools, rigorously examine licensure applicants, and sanction individual or institutional violators need to be founded upon the force of state law.

In Part II, Flexner looks at each medical school, "arranged alphabetically by states and provinces and separately characterized" (p. 183). He supplies each state's population, its number of physicians, the physician/population ratio, and the number of medical schools. For each medical school, he lists entrance requirements, attendance, teaching staff, resources available for maintenance, laboratory facilities, clinical facilities, and the date of his visit. As in Part I, Flexner names names, and does not hold back from criticizing schools (often in vivid language) for all manner of shortcomings. Neither Arkansas school "has a single redeeming feature. It is incredible that the state university should permit its name to shelter one of them" (p. 188). He reveals that the dissecting room of Kansas Medical College "was simultaneously used as a chicken yard" (p. 227). The College of Physicians and Surgeons in Boston should be "wiped out" (p. 262).

On the other hand, Minnesota is given credit for establishing a powerful state board, and centralizing medical education in the state university, while the medical school in Pittsburgh is praised for having "undergone a complete transformation" (p. 297) since its acquisition by the University of Pittsburgh. In an Appendix, Flexner provides a summary table that lists the number of professors and other instructors, the number of students, the fee income, and the annual budget (when available) by school within each state.

The Flexner Report provides a comprehensive look at turn-of-the-century physician training, and the rationale for major reforms that were eventually enacted nationally. More than any other document, it established what we now call medical education. It is also quite readable. For any scholar of (or policymaker in) medical education, this volume is simply indispensable.

35. Flexner, Abraham. *I Remember: The Autobiography of Abraham Flexner*. New York, NY: Simon and Schuster, 1940.

This work outlines the life and times of one of the most influential figures in American medical history. Flexner's account (four hundred pages long, divided into twenty-nine chapters) covers his entire life. Naturally, it pays a great deal of attention to his research into U.S. and Canadian medical education, which culminated in the production of the highly influential "Flexner Report".

As Flexner's account indicates, the activities of the American Medical Association played a major part in the development of his own research project into medical education. Dr. Henry S. Pritchett, President of the Carnegie Foundation for the Advancement of Teaching, had contacted the AMA's Council on Education concerning the project, and in fact asked Flexner "whether it might not be wise for me to have an advisory committee of physicians in studying the subject. . . . An advisory committee would, as a matter of fact, have proved a great source of embarrassment. Fortunately, both he and I forgot all about it" (p. 114).

Before he began his research, Flexner went to Chicago to consult with the Secretary of the AMA, George H. Simmons, and read the reports that the AMA Council on Medical Education had already produced. Flexner terms these reports "credible and painstaking" (p. 114). He gives the AMA (in particular, the secretary of its Council,

N.P. Colwell) much credit for carrying out reform efforts well before he did his own famous explorations.

As Flexner points out, his own report completed after eighteen months of work and published in 1910, had an immediate and powerful impact upon the debate over medical school reform. Passions ran so high that the author received anonymous death threats before discussing the report at a Chicago meeting to the AMA Council on Medical Education. Fortunately, none of the threats materialized.

36. King, Lester S. *Transformations in American Medicine.* Baltimore, MD: Johns Hopkins University Press, 1991.

In this recent work, Lester King, an eminent scholar of medical history and prominent member of the American Medical Association, examines a number of clinical breakthroughs in American medicine, and the medical researchers that made them possible. In ten chapters, Dr. King covers medical research from the eighteenth century until 1912, covering such episodes as "the discrimination of typhoid fever" and germ theory. The impact of the AMA on medical evolution is also touched upon.

Beginning in Chapter 8 ("Changing Aspects of Scientific Medicine, 1800-1850"), Dr. King steps back from the historical details and attempts to interpret what the results of "the transformation of American medicine" actually were. The growing identification of medicine as a "scientific" discipline had social implications as well. It led, for better and for worse, to an elitism--a conviction that "scientists" would know better than the common folk how to develop medical education and practice.

In King's view, this elitism had ideological and economic motivations. In addition to forming a scientific priesthood for physicians, the American Medical Association, formed in 1847, desired to control access to the profession. Like any trade union, it wished to enhance the economic well-being of its members by restricting supply. The claim of special scientific habits of thought, while true, could be used for acquiring greater social and economic power as well as additional clinical insights. Through such mechanisms as its code of ethics (which forbade contacts with any "irregular" practitioners), "the AMA had set itself up as an elite group that wanted to preserve its ideological purity . . . and incidentally to promote its own economic security" (p. 211). King outlines the dispute over medical ethics between the AMA and the American Association of Physicians that resulted.

37. Klaw, Spencer. *The Great American Medicine Show.* New York, NY: The Viking Press, 1975.

Spencer Klaw subtitles his book "The Unhealthy State of U.S. Medical Care, and What Can Be Done About It." On the whole, this substantial work (sixteen chapters and about 275 text pages) is critical of the physician profession. (However, the author takes the time to express his admiration for doctors in an introductory note.) The American Medical Association is singled out for commentary in the general indictment of the current U.S. health care system.

Mr. Klaw concludes that the AMA has inflated doctors' incomes through controls on the physician supply from medical schools. Since Flexner-era reforms, the AMA has "had the power to restrict the production of new doctors to a level that would ensure plenty of work for everyone" (p. 21). Yet the AMA control over physician education and practice has not led to effective protection of the public from incompetent or dishonest doctors. The AMA excuses its inaction on the grounds that physician policing is the task of state and county medical societies (which are also relatively inactive on this front). The AMA code of ethics is largely inoperative, according to the author.

In "The Lingering Odor of Snake Oil" (Chapter 7), Klaw describes the political and economic alliance between the AMA and the pharmaceutical industry--an alliance which he feels precludes objective consideration of drugs' effectiveness and safety by prescribing doctors. The author points out that a large portion of the AMA's income comes from pharmaceutical industry advertising in AMA publications.

The AMA is also faulted for its long-time opposition (only recently softened) toward prepaid group practice and HMOs, and its fervent efforts to forestall the adoption of Medicare in 1965. Yet, the AMA and its members have sufficiently recovered from their defeats on both fronts to wind up making substantial incomes from both of these system reforms.

Klaw recounts the gradual retreat of the AMA on national health insurance as well, pointing out that by 1969 the Association had in fact put forth its own NHI proposal. However, in the author's view, the AMA proposal would be extremely inflationary, since it preserves the doctor's "freedom" to decide what his or her own fees should be. "But even though the AMA's views have come to strike a great many Americans as archaic and self-serving, they still carry a lot of weight in Washington" (p. 227). Klaw goes on to recount the activity and successes of the American Medical Political Action Committee in the Seventies, and pessimistically concludes that its power, as part of a coalition with other powerful medical care interests (in particular, drug manufacturers and insurance companies) will preclude the enaction of a truly effective national health insurance program for some time to come.

38. Richmond, Julius B. *Currents in American Medicine.* Cambridge, MA: Harvard University Press, 1969.

Julius Richmond has compiled a very concise and short historical analysis of the evolution of medical services, education, and policy in the United States since 1900. This book was written for the "general reader" but gives some great insight to the role the AMA played in the development of today's health care system.

Beginning with the Educational Revolution in the early 1900s to the developing complexities of health care in the late sixties, Richmond presents a historical account of the AMA as a "crusading organization"(p. 5) in the 1920s to a "political-economic organization" p. 50) in the 1960s. He complains in the conclusion that the leaders of this country have the best resources in the world (organizations such as the AMA) to make educated decisions but that they are afraid their solutions may not solve the problems of the health care system.

39. Schartz, Harry. *The Case for American Medicine.* New York, NY: David McKay Company, Inc., 1972.

In this 230-page publication Harry Schartz takes, as the subtitle denotes, "A Realistic Look at Our Health Care System." As his past publications indicate, Mr. Schartz is a domestic policy analyst of not only the United States but other countries as well. In eight chapters he discusses how the American Medical System has operated up to the early seventies and voices some specific concerns over this system.

Schartz presents that American physicians and medical researchers have catapulted the American health care system to great heights as world leaders in the medical fields. There is discussion of the major concerns critics in the 1960s had of the system but he claims them as "an attack that too often leaves the high road of reasoned criticism and descends to emotionalism and misrepresentation" (p. 7).

Schartz references the AMA many times in the opening chapters for sources of statistical data. He points out the support the AMA gave to the migration of foreign trained physicians to the United States by facilitating the liberalization of immigration laws. Another major point by the author concerns the period in 1970 when Congress was enacting legislation to limit fees to physicians based on income levels in the economy. The AMA originally fought this legislation but ultimately retreated. The explanation to members was that "it was not a trade union" (p. 108) and could not negotiate fee levels because that would be in violation of anti-trust laws since all members were in actuality independent contractors and the act would be price fixing.

Mr. Schartz concludes with concerns of the deteriorating educational system and the medical research mechanism. He fears that the world class status of the U.S. will be reversed. The best road for the U.S. to take, according to Schartz, is a concentration on preventive measures and a commitment to lifestyle changes. He states we can gain "better health and greater longevity for Americans" (p. 229) by increasing the choices of health care providers, not by collectivizing American Medicine.

40. Starr, Paul. *The Social Transformation of American Medicine.* New York, NY: Basic Books, Inc., 1982.

This work, which won the author the 1984 Pulitzer Prize for general non-fiction, is intended to be "an integrated account of the social and economic development of medicine in America" (p. x). In two parts (books) that total almost 450 pages, Starr provides a chronological history of the rise of modern medicine, including the rise of the physician as the central professional force, and the hospital as the primary service delivery site, in U.S. health care. In the Introduction, entitled "The Social Origins of Professional Sovereignty", the author states the central organizing thesis of his text, that "the history of American medicine has been written as an epic of progress, but it is also a tale of social and economic conflict over the emergence of new hierarchies of power and authority, new markets, and new conditions of belief and experience" (p. 4). Starr wishes to show how politics (broadly construed) has led to our current health care system.

Starr points out that the American Medical Association "owed its impetus to the discontent felt by younger, less established doctors" (p. 90), not the most prominent physicians of the time. For a half century, the AMA had only a marginal impact on American medical education and practice. It was a poorly financed and organized society, with constant personality conflicts within the leadership. Its early attempts to forge unity among physicians were largely unsuccessful.

A chief goal of the AMA in the latter part of the nineteenth century was to eliminate the diversity of medical practice and philosophy among American physicians, and to establish a uniform, science-based profession in its place. Indeed, "as long as physicians were divided, any move by the regulars to bring back licensing or reform medical education seemed like a narrow maneuver on their part aimed at winning advantage over the dissenters" (p. 99). Attempts at compromise with the medical sects led to further divisions within the

AMA. The urbanization of the U.S. and further advances in medical science, however, steadily tilted the balance of power toward the orthodox physicians within the AMA. Gradually, licensing control was extended in state after state in the 1890-1910 period. The AMA gained additional strength through reorganization from the county level up, with a revitalization of state medical societies (and corresponding increases in influence over state governments).

By 1920, sixty percent of American physicians belonged to the AMA. "In a remarkably short time, physicians began to achieve the unity and coherence that had so long eluded them. . . . From this period dates the power of what came to be called organized medicine" (p. 110). The Flexner Report and subsequent changes in state laws regarding medical education and practice gave the AMA substantial control over American health care.

The AMA further consolidated physician control by effectively opposing the development of corporate enterprises in health care. Though this was portrayed by the Association as a defense of medical idealism against capitalist money-grubbing, it was in fact the establishment of a physician monopoly, and an avoidance of the characteristic hierarchical control of modern industry. Only physicians would be permitted to profit from health care.

In a developing capitalist democracy, however, such victories are never permanent. In particular, the Great Depression, and the rise of the New Deal and Franklin Roosevelt in the 1930s, cast doubt upon the physicians' contentions that their professional interests coincided with the larger interests of the public when it came to health care organization. From then on, physicians and the AMA had to fight pitched battles with those who would subordinate their authority to that of government and/or the corporate sector through one form or another of restructured health services delivery combined with insurance. Physicians, led by the AMA, successfully forestalled many such efforts in the Forties and Fifties, but private health insurance programs continued to expand. The marriage of science to medicine meant large-scale government funding--which led to increased public controls. The passage of Medicare and Medicaid, which ignited the ongoing cost inflation in health care that now preoccupies the nation, meant the end of the unique controlling "mandate" that physicians possessed. The Seventies and Eighties would see "The Coming of the Corporation" to health care, and the steady reduction of physicians into employees.

In Starr's view, it will be difficult for the AMA to retain its influence within this environment. "'We are not opposed to the corporate practice of medicine,' says Dr. Sammons of the AMA. 'There is no way we could be' . . . The growth of corporate medicine has simply gone too far for the AMA to oppose it outright" (p. 446).

41. Stevens, Rosemary. *American Medicine and the Public Interest.* New Haven, CT: Yale University Press, 1971.

This massive (over five hundred text pages) work is intended to be a comprehensive examination of the history of American health care since colonial times, with a particular emphasis on the impact of professional specialization. Dr. Stevens, a Professor in the School of Medicine at Yale University, divides her work into five parts: The Professional Setting; Formal Recognition of the Specialties, 1900-1930; The Specialties Come of Age, 1930-1950; Professional Structures Reexamined; and The Medical Profession and Medical Care.

The author gives due attention to the various roles that the American Medical Association has played within U.S. health care. In Chapter 3 ("Reform Achieved: The AMA and Medical Education, 1890-1914"), Dr. Stevens gives the AMA credit for being the primary "catalyst for reform" (p. 60), though she does feel that the AMA efforts led to increased elitism and racial exclusivity as well as clinical excellence. Within the first three chapters, she provides a fairly detailed and standard history of the rise and development of the Association, including the establishment of its flagship Journal.

In later chapters, AMA activities are extensively reported, and intertwined with the general development of the U.S. health care system. In Stevens' narrative, they show a powerful but increasingly reactionary organization. AMA political activism is almost entirely focused on the need to forestall national government intervention (particularly in the form of national health insurance), and the preservation of the fee-for-service status quo. The defeat over Medicare in 1965 ended an era of AMA dominance.

However, Dr. Stevens does not confuse the end of AMA dominance with a loss of effective political power. According to her, "present signs are that the AMA will become less of a spokesman for medical education and manpower development . . . less of a trade association . . . and more of a negotiating body with government, and a governmental agent. In so doing, its power will be strengthened" (p. 532). Unlike some other scholars, Dr. Stevens sees increasing governmental involvement in health care (even including national health insurance), as augmenting the power of the AMA and other organized medical groups. "Increasing organization of governmental programs means increasing organization of the medical profession" (p. 532).

(B) Articles

42. Berliner, Howard S. "New Light in the Flexner Report: Notes on the AMA - Carnegie Foundation Background." *Bulletin of the History of Medicine* (1977): 603-604.

The author, having researched newly released files of 1907-1910 from the Carnegie Foundation, Library of Congress, and the AMA, provides highly interesting insight to the Flexner Report. Berliner confirms that reform of medical education was already proceeding rapidly through self-reform efforts of the profession - well before Flexner's survey. The author maintains that the Carnegie Foundation's motivation is helping the AMA evaluate medical schools fostering social stability; they sought to strengthen the middle class and ameliorate class antagonisms between the urban proletariat and capitalist upper class. The foundation believed that better educated and financially secure doctors, lawyers, engineers and other professionals would provide that buffer and help stabilize society. The AMA, on the other hand, sought a reduction in the surplus of doctors as well as more scientifically educated physicians who would regain professional respect from the public and earn a more lucrative income.

The article also relates how Abraham Flexner was selected to conduct the survey through brotherly influence, how many doubted his judgment and "somewhat erratic tendencies," and how Flexner relied so heavily upon the Rockefeller Institutes' recommendations for medical education drafted in 1907.

Berliner concludes that it was not the Flexner Report which, by itself, changed medical education, but the money poured into medical education by large philanthropic foundations between 1910 and the 1930s.

43. Ellman, Michael H. "William Crawford Gorgas and the AMA." *Journal of the American Medical Association* 243(7) (February 15, 1980): 659-660.

This brief article chronicles the story of how the AMA supported Dr. William Gorgas in combating yellow fever and malaria through sanitation measures that helped insure completion of the Panama Canal Zone. The physicians' military superiors did not support Gorgas' measures in Panama until the AMA arranged for an investigation of health problems and helped get Gorgas appointed to the Canal Commission in 1907. This AMA support put Gorgas in the position to eliminate yellow fever and halve the malaria rate. Dr. Gorgas served as President of the AMA in 1909 and became Surgeon General of the U.S.

Army in 1914 where he reshaped the Medical Corps and got it ready for World War I.

44. Frederickson, Donald S. "The National Institutes of Health, Yesterday, Today and Tomorrow." *Public Health Reports* 93 (1978): 642-647.

The author, as Director of the National Institutes of Health (NIH), provides a short history of this important institution since 1930. Frederickson accounts its specialty centers from its original charter in nutrition and microbiology for the Public Health Service. The author shows that the NIH greatly benefited from the general post-W.W.II assumption by the federal government of the funding for scientific research. Like the Atomic Energy and Space Flight Programs, medical research received major increases in federal funding during the late 1940's, 1950's and early 60's.

Frederickson maintains that by 1963 the U.S. was pre-eminent in biomedical research. Support went to foreign as well as domestic research programs. In the process, Congress became more directly involved in setting research priorities. From 1938 until 1974, specialty institutes, General Medical Science and a National Library of Medicine were created to tackle cancer, heart disease, infectious diseases, eyes, environmental problems, and aging. The emphasis in the process is to safeguard against political misuse (e.g., genetic engineering) while ensuring research is translated as rapidly as possible into practical, useful applications.

45. Harris, Richard. "Medicare, Part III-We Do Not Compromise." *The New Yorker* (July 16, 1966): 11-17.

This lengthy article is the third in a series of four articles on Medicare. Harris details the political battles waged intensively by the AMA and others, hoping to preclude passage of this major health program. The article covers the period from the early 1950s to 1965, from immediately before previous efforts under Presidents Truman and Kennedy, to passage of the bill under President Johnson. The author maintains that the AMA, in making the issue known to millions of Americans who were not aware of its magnitude and implications, "accomplished something it had never intended--it stirred up a great national debate." Harris covers the 1960 Kerr-Mills bill which provided Welfare aid and served as a poor compromise in lieu of an insurance program. This compromise allowed many Congressmen to avoid loss of supporters during the 1960 elections. The bill, however, needed strong state funding to match federal revenues and, in the end, did not significantly expand coverage to the needy.

Harris then details AMA actions to influence the 1962 and 1964 elections, in the process of combating the Medicare bill. He points out the limited impact these actions had on voting outcome and shows that many successfully elected Congressmen were promoting Medicare. Of particular interest in this article is the section on AMA's 1963 decision to refrain from joining in with the Surgeon General in citing tobacco smoking as injurious to personal health. Harris accounts this purported appeasement of the tobacco state Senators in hopeful exchange of winning their vote against Medicare. The article furthermore includes the origin and actions of the American Medical Political Action Committee (AMPAC).

46. Henderson, Elmer L. "The Responsibility of American Medicine." *Journal of the American Medical Association* 143 (1950): 783-785.

Dr. Henderson, as the new AMA President, addresses his association with a rallying cry to keep America free from becoming a "socialist state". This address serves as an excellent example of how the AMA interpreted advocacy of compulsory health insurance as just one of the many indicators that Washington bureaucrats support a welfare state at the expense of individual socioeconomic and political freedoms. Dr. Henderson accounts the great progress made by medicine due to the AMA since the turn of the century. He then forecasts major accomplishments in health care for the future. Henderson believes that this progress is seriously threatened by the chance of socialism in America.

47. King, Lester S. "The Flexner Report of 1910." *Journal of the American Medical Association* (1983): 88-95.

Dr. King describes the Flexner Report on medical education as "probably the most grossly overrated document in American medical history,"...a report endowed "with canonical status that has resulted in some horrendous distortion of the historical record." After that eye opening start, the author shows that problems and recommended solutions for American medical schools were already well documented and many were being acted upon. Specifically, the better medical schools were starting to require 1 or 2 years of college before entry to medical school. Physical sciences and clinical methods were also being strengthened in the curriculum. State medical boards were beginning to raise standards for licensing and many of the poorer schools were folding up under financial pressure. Dr. King documents how the AMA's Council on Medical Education, founded in 1904, had already begun its own surveys and ratings of schools, and was calling for specific reforms and endowment by wealthy philanthropers.

Dr. King then accounts how the AMA approached the Carnegie Foundation in 1908 and asked Foundation President Henry S. Pritchett to investigate and publish a special report on medical education. Such action would provide an outside, objective critique of existing schools and draw publicity and hopefully endowment monies for raising standards.

The author also documents how the AMA participated in the Flexner whirlwind in the school inspections and how the report helped to provide the attention, impetus and funding to continue reforms already called for by the AMA and begun by the better schools. This historical vignette is an excellent and highly interesting account of a major event in the U.S. history of organized medicine.

48. Kotelchuck, Ronda. "The Depression and the American Medical Association." *Health PAC Bulletin* 69 (March/April 1976): 13-18.

This is an excellent article addressing the impact of the Great Depression on organized medicine, hospitals, individual physicians and related elements. Kotelchuck shows how economic crises often act to accelerate historic trends already underway and to intensify the pressure for social and political change." In this case, the Depression accelerated processes which threatened private practice, augmented the role of government, saw the rise and enormous impact of medical insurance, and led to the specialization, centralization and corporation of health care. The author includes the AMA's response to a perceived doctor surplus, its apprehension of growing public health programs like public immunization, its battle against including national health insurance in the 1935 Social Security Act, and its resistance to group medical practice or corporate medicine. Kotelchuck also shows the major impact of the Depression on hospitals, such as federal funding of Public Works Administration programs to build over 1,000 new public hospital buildings, and follow-up construction by the Works Progress Administration. Finally, the author accounts the growth of Blue Cross which rescued so many hospitals from financial ruin, yet also postponed the advent of national health insurance.

49. Mayer, Milton. "The Rise and Fall of Dr. Fishbein." *Harper's Magazine* (1949): 76-85

This article provides an account of Dr. Morris Fishbein's 37 years with AMA and his work as Editor of the Association's journals (JAMA). Mayer first underlines the importance of JAMA in financing most AMA activities: in 1948, the Journal netted a nontaxable $1,400,000 and was truly the "heart of AMA". JAMA's Seal of Acceptance meant profits for manufacturers and, for the AMA, lucrative ads placed in the Journal. Mayer paints the picture of a very proud, strong-willed editor who well understood the power of the pen. Fishbein, moreover, was a prolific author as well as public speaker. His history of the AMA's first hundred years is a true classic. In the end, it was Fishbein's overzealous actions such as his war against national insurance (i.e. socialized medicine) that led to his dismissal. Mayer's article provides a highly interesting treatment of a most influential and controversial figure of organized medicine.

50. Numbers, Ronald L. "Organized Medicine Didn't Always Oppose NHI." *Hospital Progress* (July 1978): 6, 10, 16.

Dr. Numbers, as Chairman of the Department of the History of Medicine of the University of Wisconsin, provides this summary of compulsory health insurance and organized medicine. Numbers traces the origin of efforts to provide national legislation and how the AMA promoted these efforts from 1916 to 1920. The author accounts the influence of German and British insurance acts and the belief by many physicians that NHI would raise their incomes and was inevitably coming anyway. Then, a series of factors helped reverse this supportive stance. U.S. entry into World War I in April 1917 interrupted the general social reform movement and brought in anti-German hysteria. The October 1917 Bolshevik revolution then frightened Americans with socialism. Furthermore, individual states began voting against expanded health insurance, removing the attitude that NHI was a given fact. Overall, however, the foremost cause for a reversal of opinion was the early experience with workers compensation insurance and the new belief that NHI would actually decrease physician income. Dr. Numbers concludes with the conclusion that the campaign promoting NHI until 1920 in effect created lasting suspicion and opposition to legislation for even voluntary coverage, well into the twentieth century.

51. Strickland, Stephen P. "Integration of Medical Research and Health Policies." *Science* 173 (September 17, 1971): 1093-1103.

This lengthy article, by a Washington-based health and education program consultant, traces U.S. government policy and funding for medical research since the 1940s. Strickland documents the enormous increase in budgets for the National Institutes of Health and the Congressional role in advancing basic research and its vision of eliminatory disease. The article maintains that the AMA's preoccupation with opposing national health insurance allowed the government to rapidly enter the medical research support business without opposition from organized medicine. Strickland additionally assesses the results of government funded medical research. The author says it succeeded in creating a national biomedical research network and led to the U.S. becoming the leader in biomedical science. This, in turn, "revolutionized the range of diagnostic, therapeutic and preventive capabilities of medicine." Regarding its impact in medical schools, however, Strickland says the funding led to enormous growth in faculties and facilities but had little effect on the creation of more doctors. To the contrary, the federal government intentionally held back on funding student grants, loans and direct funding of medical school operations. Regarding this matter, AMA's chairman of the Board of Trustees, Louis H. Baver, cautioned that the proposal to support medical schools with federal funds "would give the government a foot in the door... for federal control of medical education."

Nevertheless, Congress took a first, small step to directly support medical and paramedical education in 1963; the Health Professions Education Assistance Act provided grants for facilities construction and student loans. This support was broadened through the Health Manpower Act of 1968 and other support. By comparison, however, federal funding continued to emphasize medical research rather than assistance to medical students. Moreover, Strickland concludes by underlying the necessity for the federal government to develop a more comprehensive, integrated policy for solving our health care problems centered on costs, coverage and related factors.

52. White, Philip L. "A Brief History of the American Medical Association's Council in Foods and Nutrition." *Nutrition Today* (January/February 1975): 10-13.

The author, Secretary of the AMA's Council on Foods and Nutrition, accounts the Council's beginning, purpose and major accomplishments from 1929 until 1975. The article documents the council's work in evaluating food products and vitamins for nutritional value and validity of advertising claims. The council assisted government regulators to develop legislation revising the Food, Drug and Cosmetic Act, and advised government officials on such matters as combating malnutrition was most successful in fostering research the council on nutrition, the teaching of nutrition in medical schools and hospitals, and the production of monographs, articles, books and synopses to exchange and discriminate knowledge on nutrition. It presented awards for outstanding contributions in clinical nutrition and provided medical student research fellowships. Advisory support was provided key members of the food industry, with special attention paid to special purpose food such as for babies. In 1975, the Council was placed on inactive status due to fiscal constraints, with the AMA's Department of Foods and Nutrition assuming responsibilities for its programs.

53. Wilsford, David. "The Cohesion and Fragmentation of Organized Medicine in France and the U.S." *Journal of Health Politics, Policy and Law* 12(3) (Fall 1987): 481-503.

The author contrasts French and American medical professions and summarized why American organized medicine is more cohesive and politically and economically successful in its contests with government employees and insurers. Mr. Wilsford attributes the strength of American organized medicine to its tendency to organize "universally", better accommodating divergent interests of physicians. The author also addresses factors of fragmentation threatening organized medicine and how rising health care costs have increased government intervention. The author addresses factors of medical profession, cohesion such as common medical training, ethics, public esteem, regular contact and the role of the AMA. The article provides an excellent review of AMA's actions in medical education, gatekeeping of physician production, accreditation, linking membership with hospital privileges, offering group insurance, and providing professional journals. Mr. Wilsford points out the lack of competition to the AMA from counterpart associations and gives examples of how AMA coopted dissident movements in order to remain strong. Wilsford's treatment of the results stemming from AMA reforms of 1901 and 1903 is especially well done. Wilsford does include the fact that AMA is not all-powerful, in that less than half of U.S. physicians are members and that factors like the growing number of salaried physicians offer new challenges to organizational unity in many issues.

54. Worthington, W. Curtis. "A Study in Post-Flexner Survival: The Medical College of the State of South Carolina, 1913." *Journal of the American Medical Association* 266(7) (August 21, 1991): 981-984.

This is a fascinating article about the challenges and accomplishments of a medical college that survived an unfavorable review by Abraham Flexner. The report described the college as having "traditions and a certain present dignity" but was highly critical of its "poor physical facilities, lack of full-time faculty, lack of equipment, and lack of money" (p.981).

After tracing the survival and success of the medical school as it overcame the Flexner indictment, the author concludes, "As these events illustrate, the public good often rests on a wide variety of seemingly unrelated forces, chance events, incompatible players, and unlikely associations" (p. 984).

5

THE AMA MISSION, ORGANIZATION AND INFLUENCE

The AMA's rise to preeminence in the twentieth century was significantly linked to its elaborate but decentralized organizational structure. National leadership, as represented in the House of Delegates, could act decisively. But with a base of strength in the medical societies at the state and county levels, enough autonomy was preserved to allow for regional and local variations. However, these structural developments did not prevent serious conflicts over policy to develop among AMA membership. Despite an overall consensus, the proportion of American physicians holding AMA membership steadily declined, until the Association formally represented less than fifty percent of physicians by the 1980s.

In political terms, the American Medical Association has been one of the most spectacularly successful interest groups in the history of the United States. However sincerely idealistic the AMA and its membership may have been (and are) in working for higher quality medical education and practice, the fact is that no other occupational group has ever gained such effective control over an entire industry of such central importance. Even as AMA and physician power erode during the eighties, American doctors are still on average the wealthiest professionals in history, with enormous control over their workplace and major influence over public policy at all levels.

The books and articles here provide a wide range of interpretations of AMA political activity, and how the Association has influenced other organizations and social institutions. Social scientists emphasize how the AMA's organization, combined with the financial resources at its disposal, have led to major political influence. The cohesiveness of

AMA membership, as well as a working consensus on professional and political interests, have aided the Association in wielding its power. They also point out that the AMA has excelled at forming effective coalitions with other organizations (hospital associations, business interests, and, at times, political parties) when required, and has been aided by the generally positive image that physicians have in the mind of the American public. They are also objective enough to point to the AMA's political weaknesses as well as its strengths, noting a gradual decline in the organization's effectiveness during the latter half of this century.

Partisan commentators provide widely differing interpretations of AMA motivations and behavior. Both sympathizers and opponents often overstate the Association's impact and influence. Those approving of AMA activities point to the undeniable benefits of AMA concern for quality health care and education, and assert that Association power has been used to serve the best interests of patients. On the other hand, authors who are critical of the AMA note that the organization's members have done quite well by doing good--preserving a service monopoly and skewing the distribution of resources within the health care system. A number portray the organization as a monument to greed and insensitivity to social needs, the chief obstacle to a truly humane system of health care in the U.S.

Though some of the portraits are caricatures of AMA good and evil, most of the authors examined here begin with the assumption that the AMA has been an extraordinarily influential organization, responsible for shaping modern American health care. They differ on the whys and hows of this influence. They also disagree about the effects of Association power on the U.S. health care sector, and American society as a whole.

(A) Books

55. Ehrenreich, Barbara, and John Ehrenreich. *The American Health Empire*. New York, NY: Random House, 1970.

"If this book can be said to have a single thesis, it is that the American health system is not in business for people's health" (p. vii). The authors, noted and outspoken political liberals, are members of the Health Policy Advisory Center (Health-PAC), a New York City-based advocacy group. They see the U.S. health care system as dominated by professional elites that primarily work for the best interests of American capitalism and the economic upper classes. They call for "radical social change"--the democratic restructuring of health care.

The titles of the nineteen chapters of the book ("The Blue Cross We Bear", "Medicaid: Killers of the Dream", and "The Empire Has No Clothes") clearly express their viewpoint.

The American Medical Association is portrayed as the chief power center for elitist and plutocratic health policy in the "medical-industrial complex", and a major obstacle to rationalizing the health care system. The AMA prevents medical school expansion, thus contributing to the shortage of doctors. However, the authors also suggest that the Association's power was at its highest in the Forties and Fifties. Now the AMA has lost political influence to other elements of the medical elite--hospitals, equipment and pharmaceutical companies, and insurers, in particular. The era of the physician, and the AMA, is coming to an end. "The battles go on, but the war is over. . . . While the AMA pours its money into symbolic battles and public relations face-lifting, the empires are steadily, confidently building. There is no going back for the American health care system . . . . The age of the guild-dominated, individual medical craftsman is over" (p.39).

The authors elsewhere refer to the AMA's political efforts as "pathetic" and "rear-guard" (p. 48). They claim that initiatives produced by the Association tend to be defensive in nature, and are offered to preclude more effective and systemic reforms. (The AMA proposals for national health insurance fall into this category.)

56. Feldstein, Paul J. *Health Associations and the Demand for Legislation.* Cambridge, MA: Ballinger Publishing Co., 1977.

This book, authored by an eminent political economist at the University of Michigan, explores the ways in which health associations exert their influence to promote the enaction of health legislation by federal and state legislatures. Chapter One provides a model of the demand for health legislation, based on an interest group theory of political behavior. Chapters Two through Seven provide studies of how seven different associations (the American Medical Association, the American Dental Association, the American Nurses' Association, the American Hospital Association, Blue Cross, the Association of American Medical Colleges, and the American Association of Dental Schools) operate in the political arena to attain their goals.

In Chapter Two ("The American Medical Association"), Feldstein states that the AMA is "the most influential of the health professional associations" (p. 27), and a role model for more recently formed groups. It is true that the AMA has suffered a steady decline in its membership in recent years--partly because of greater physician specialization (and consequent attention to specialist associations), and partly because nonmember doctors can in fact reap the benefits of many AMA activities (the "free-rider" problem). Nevertheless, the AMA has been generally effective in the policymaking process. The author provides a brief historical description of AMA political activities, including efforts to defeat national health insurance proposals in the 1930s and 1940s, lobbying against the enaction of Medicare in 1965, and attempts to prevent the establishment of Professional Standard Review Organizations (PSROs) in the Seventies. According to Feldstein, "the AMA seeks legislative activity on both the supply side, to restrict the number of physicians, and on the demand side, to increase the demand for physician services and to secure as high a fee as possible for those services" (p. 35).

To maximize the power of physicians, the AMA has also worked to provide doctors with effective control over the complements to physicians' services, such as hospitals and other health care professionals (nurses and allied health personnel). The Association has consistently endeavored to prevent the use of physician substitutes--osteopaths, chiropractors and optometrists. Finally, the AMA has focused on restricting the supply of physicians through control over licensure and accreditation procedures, and barriers to Foreign Medical Graduate (FMG) immigration.

In "Concluding Comments" (Chapter Eight), Feldstein suggests that politically successful medical associations (the AMA in particular) have significantly contributed to increased costs and decreased innovation and efficiency within the health care system, primarily by restricting competition. To advance the public's interests, he concludes that the political power of health associations will have to be curbed, and the health care system opened up to greater levels of competition.

57. Feldstein, Paul, J. *The Politics of Health Legislation.* Ann Arbor, MI: Health Administration Press, 1988.

The relationship between legislative politics and health policy is the subject of this book. Paul J. Feldstein is Professor and FHP Foundation Distinguished Chair in Health Care Management at the Graduate School of Management, University of California at Irvine. In a relatively short (about 250 pages, in ten chapters) text, he uses concepts from economic theory to develop an "economic self-interest" model of legislative policymaking. He then uses the model to explain how the American Medical Association and other health care interest groups get favorable legislation enacted, and how such statutes have historically affected the health care environment.

According to Feldstein, AMA political influence peaked in the late Forties and early Fifties. The enaction of Medicare in 1965 was viewed as a major defeat for the organization, but the details of the legislation actually resulted in great benefits for physicians. Until the late Sixties "the AMA was able to overcome the potentially divisive issue of specialty societies by understanding and representing the common economic interests of all physicians; the maintenance of fee-for-service practice without government interference"(p. 42).

More recently, the AMA has attempted to maintain broad-based support from the increasingly diverse population of American physicians by adding public health concerns (such as seat-belt usage and tobacco subsidies) to its more traditional economic issues. But the organization continues to have problems with "free rider" physicians, who benefit from AMA legislative efforts without becoming members (preferring to focus on relevant specialty societies instead). In the Seventies and Eighties, AMA policy activities have produced mixed results. AMA-sponsored increases in residency requirements have provided low-cost complementary labor while deferring additional competition. On the other hand, prospective payment systems have been enacted over AMA opposition, and FTC antitrust regulations have been applied to physician activities.

58. Gilb, Corinne Lathrop. *Hidden Hierarchies: The Professions and Government.* New York: Harper and Row, 1966.

This is a fascinating treatise on the role of professions in shaping governmental policymaking. In essence the professions are seen as a subgovernment system that serve to meet and occasionally exploit the will of the people in society. The influence of large and powerful associations such as the AMA, ABA, and NEA are well documented with numerous examples of their influence and impact on government. The AMA's role in shaping insurance regulatory policy, hospital accreditation, minority issues, judicial review, medical education, ethics, and many other areas of public policy is described. The book also provides several tables and charts with data that provide a clear picture of professional dominance in American society.

In the final analysis, the question of the predominate mode of policymaking is raised. The reader must choose from one of the following: democracy, bureaucracy, or oligarchy. The author makes a strong argument that the American political scene is one that is heavily shaped by a professional oligarchy with each association serving to meet the needs for democratic process through their own internal politics.

59. Ginzberg, Eli. *The Limits of Health Reform.* New York, NY: Basic Books, Inc., 1977.

This work is a continuation of Dr. Ginzberg's long-standing analysis of current U.S. health care policy, and possibilities for reform and improvement. On this occasion, the eminent scholar's work through the Conservation of Human Resources program at Columbia University was supported by grants from the Robert Wood Johnson Foundation and the U.S. Department of Labor.

The twelve-chapter text (with two hundred text pages) is divided into three parts: "Framework", "Goals" and "Prospects for Reform". In Chapter Three ("The Postwar Experience"), Dr. Ginzberg briefly outlines American Medical Association opposition to national health insurance during the 1930-1950 period--opposition that successfully forestalled enaction of health insurance proposals advocated by the Roosevelt and Truman Administrations. In the same chapter, he also discusses AMA opposition to federal subsidies for medical schools and governmentally-sponsored expansion of medical school enrollments. However, the AMA has cooperated with the Medicare program "once it was assured that the new legislation would not be used to disturb existing relationships between physicians and their patients" (p. 31).

Within Ginzberg's narrative, there are also brief references to AMA opposition to HMOs (now lessened) and the admission of foreign medical graduates. The author concludes that AMA political power is now on the decline, given the rise of active specialty societies and falling AMA membership rolls. Nevertheless, the Association "retains considerable clout. It still is able to beat back most attempts that aim to alter the long-standing relations between physician and patient, to restrict the rights of the profession to practice according to its own goals, or to weaken its economic position" (p. 166).

60. Lewis, Charles E., Rashi Fein, and David Mechanic. *A Right to Health.* New York, NY: John Wiley & Sons, 1976.

This work, started with a grant from the Robert Wood Johnson Foundation, is subtitled "the problem of access to primary medical care". The authors (eminent and extensively-published health policy scholars) take both conceptual and historical approaches in analyzing the problems that the U.S. has had in providing access to primary health care for all of its citizens. The book (over three hundred pages long, with nineteen chapters plus appendices), concludes with a section on policy options.

The authors principally look at the role of the American Medical Association in developing primary care in "Family Practice: the

Primary Care Specialty" (Chapter 7). As they note, the AMA began efforts to develop recommendations for upgrading general practice in 1956. However, the twenty pilot family practice programs that were established as a result received inadequate support and interest, and ended in 1969. The AMA was more successful in gaining support for a family practice option when its Ad Hoc Committee on Education for Family Practice issued the Willard Report in 1966. The authors discuss the 1969 AMA recognition of the family practice specialty, and point out that the AMA and other organizations "have mounted promotional campaigns and extracurricular programs to involve students in primary care" (p. 82), and have subsequently surveyed medical schools to assess resulting changes in educational programs.

In Chapter Eight ("Efforts to Increase the Number of authors briefly touch on the AMA policy shift in favor of increasing medical school enrollment in the early sixties, including more (and more equitably distributed) primary care physicians. ". . . In 1973, the AMA president-elect included among organized medicine's priority goals an increase in primary care physicians and a better geographic distribution of health professionals, especially to deprived areas" (p. 93). They also describe the AMA physician surveys to ascertain the professional and geographic distribution of doctors.

61. Melhado, Evan M., W. Feinberg, and H. M. Swartz, Editors. *Money, Power and Health Care.* Ann Arbor, MI: Health Administration Press, 1988.

The title of this text accurately describes the overall theme of the nine articles (spanning approximately three hundred pages) within. Though they deal with a variety of substantive topics from a number of disciplinary perspectives, all of the authors are concerned with how the U.S. health care system is being transformed by deregulation and marketplace competition (money) and the determined political struggle of concerned interest groups (power). The three editors (who are also authors) are faculty members at the University of Illinois, Urbana - Champaign who focus in their research on the relationships between science, technology and public policy.

In Chapter 5 ("Consumer Sovereignty in a Competitive Market: Fact or Fiction?"), Thomas W. O'Rourke discusses "the landmark case in which the Federal Trade Commission (FTC) sued the American Medical Association (AMA) and two Connecticut medical societies" (p. 162). Ultimately, the FTC ordered the AMA to stop its efforts to restrict the advertising of physician services. However, groups such as the AMA will probably continue to oppose pro-competition health policies, and support fee-for-service medicine and cost-based reimbursement mechanisms.

According to James E. Black ("The Sentimental Marketplace: Who Controls Child Care?"), the child welfare movement of the early twentieth century had to carefully craft its proposed reforms to avoid encroaching on the occupational prerogatives of physicians (which would antagonize the AMA). "The clinical sphere of the movement was restricted to nonrenumerated, preventive measures like immunizations and hygiene instruction, and to medical care of only the very poorest children in charity hospitals" (p. 219).

Nevertheless, as Black shows, general practitioners felt threatened, and "an unusual alliance, including the AMA, chiropractors, antivaccinationists, and antisuffragists, adopted a virulently misogynistic tone in their opposition to [the Sheppard-Towner Act, a child welfare measure]" (p. 223). In 1922, the AMA House of Delegates labeled the Act "an imported socialist scheme," prompting a major conflict between the bulk of the AMA and its Pediatrics Section, which supported the legislation. Though passed, the Sheppard-Towner Act was not renewed by Congress when it was reconsidered in 1929.

In "Thirty Years of Change in Medical Education, Money and Power," Harold M. Swartz and Ann Berry Flood discuss the role of group practice, and point out that the AMA Committee on the Costs of Medical Care endorsed the concept in 1932. But in the opinion of the AMA, group practices were only to be established on grounds of economy: "the acceptable motivation to join group practice was to reduce overhead costs, and not to alter the practice of medicine" (p. 295).

62. Roemer, Milton I. and J. W. Friedman. *Doctors In Hospitals*. Baltimore, MD: The Johns Hopkins Press, 1971.

Roemer and Friedman explore the relationship of the medical staff organization to the hospital organization and define the implications. They discuss their conclusions of the effectiveness of this relationship in the performance of the hospital. The authors distinguish between "hospital performance" and "efficiency" relative to how the hospital, as a social organization, "does." They state that "from this research it is evident that advancement of the hospital toward the concept of a community center for delivery or provision of all types of health service will bear a relationship to its medical staff organization." (p.301)

In this 302 page book, the authors mention the AMA relatively few times. When they do reference the AMA, they are generally pointing out what they perceive as the organization's negative views on societal policy making. For example, the authors explain how the AMA opposed prepaid group practices and did not even allow "salaried" physicians as members to the local medical societies. Also pointed out was the AMA's opposition to close physician/hospital relations, because they feared that "corporate practice would absolutely destroy the personal responsibilities and relationships which were essential to the best interest of the patient" (p. 284). Roemer and Friedman contend that the AMA was in its earlier years much more representative of the general practitioners than it was in the 1970s.

(B) Articles

63. Baldwin, Mark. "Industry PACs Donate Thousands to 'Maintain Access' to Legislators." *Modern Healthcare* (October 24, 1986): 28.

This short article summarizes 1986 election activity by healthcare-related political action committees (PACs). Baldwin provides specific figures given by several PACs to influence to vote for or against specific congressmen.

The article also contrasts the different strategies among PACs. While the Political Action Committee of the American Hospital Association and the Federation of American Health System's PAC usually only withhold support from the campaign funds of an opponent, the AMA will spend sizable funds to unseat an "enemy." In 1986, the AMA's PAC (AMPAC) gave about $4.5 million in more than 200 electoral races nationwide. Most contributions fell between $3,500 and $5,000. AMPAC, however, spent approximately $200,000 in an unsuccessful effort to unseat Fortney Stark (D-California), a strong critic of the AMA while Chairman of the Health Subcommittee of the House Ways and Means Committee. Baldwin's article suggests that PAC funding has mixed results at best.

64. Brazda, Jerome F. "The AMA in Washington: Is it Doing Its Job?" *Impact* (June 22, 1979): 13, 15.

The author, a veteran journalist, interviewed friends and foes of the AMA to assess its political strength and accomplishments. While opinions widely vary, most see the AMA (in 1979) as a very effective lobby in Washington, and in state elections through campaign contributions to politicians by the "independent" American Medical Political Action Committee (AMPAC). Brazda provides examples of legislative battles lost by the AMA, as well as several important victories. One critic cited by the author charges the AMA is a "potent force in the shaping of health policy, but usually a negative one." Another charges the AMA is "too conservative to carry much weight in Washington," during periods when the Democrats control Congress and the White House.

65. Breo, Dennis L. "AMA's Washington Office--Its Legend and Its Legacy." *American Medical News* (June 18, 1982): 3, 12, 13-14, 36, and 38-39.

The article accounts the many battles over national health insurance, caps to physicians' fees and the Federal Trade Commission's challenge. Breo traces the differing approaches taken by the AMA to influence legislators, from using the California public relations firm of Whitaker and Baxter, to establishing AMDAC in 1961 and using aggressive state and local medical society activities to personally influence Congressmen. Breo shows that the new twelve story AMA building opened at 1101 Vermont Avenue in April 1982 reflects the AMA's decision to permanently strengthen its influence in Washington.

On the other hand, the AMA's Chairman of the Board of Trustees, Dr. Joseph F. Boyle, states that the main association headquarters will stay in Chicago symbolizing the AMA's intention to emphasize promotion of the science and art of medicine above its political activities. This Breo article is a good summary of 35 years of AMA political objectives and strategy.

66. "Building a Better AMA: Strategies for 1987 and Beyond." *Michigan Medicine* (March 1987): 128-130, 156, 160, 172, 184 and 186.

This article provides an excellent summary of newly stated AMA fundamental purposes, key objectives, strategies, needs and new initiatives to better fulfill its mission. The summary is an abridged introduction to the 1987 AMA Plan and Budget. While a thorough review of the AMA Constitution will offer details on purpose and responsibilities, this article succinctly outlines the Association's charter and how it intends to accomplish it. As stated, the AMA House of Delegates approved a new "key objective" in 1986 which is:

> "To contribute to the professional and personal development of member physicians and the betterment of the health of the public by developing and distributing information; by advocating the health

> profession as a whole where the image, expertise, and national sign of the AMA prove useful."

By acting upon these strategies, the AMA hopes to gain the active support of a majority of physicians and high levels of public trust and confidence. New initiatives are therefore designed to demonstrate the AMA's competence, objectivity and commitment to excellence in a highly visible manner to the profession and the public.

67. Capuzzi, Cecelia. "Power and Interest Groups: A study of the ANA and AMA." *Nursing Outlook* 28(8) (August 1980): 487-492.

The author reviews twelve factors that influence the power of any interest group, and then compares the status of the American Nurses Association (ANA) with the American Medical Association. Ms. Capuzzi shows the AMA to be much stronger due to having more members, greater capabilities to reward and punish members, more wealth, the professional status and importance attributed to doctors, stronger leadership, more political experience at lobbying, more inside connections, and a greater willingness to expend resources. This brief article provides a good summary of many of the key factors which have made the AMA strong.

68. Cotton, Paul. "AMPAC Change in Strategy Increases Payoff at Polls." *Medical World News* 29(23) (December 12, 1988): 31.

This article addresses the 1988 election campaign efforts by the American Medical Political Action Committee (AMPAC). Although still the largest health-related PAC, in terms of expenditures, it had fallen from its 1986 position as top PAC spender to the third overall. AMPAC spent $2.1 million in regular congressional contributions, $.9 million in independent expenditures ("shadow campaigns") and $.6 million for "research and volunteer training." AMPAC decided not to try to unseat "unfriendly" incumbents but rather to support friendlies and open races. All except one of AMPAC's shadow candidates won, and overall AMPAC expenditures were split fairly evenly between Democrats and Republicans.

69. Demkovich, Linda E. "The AMA--Reports of Its Death Have Been Greatly Exaggerated." *National Journal* (December 1, 1979): 2017, 2019-2022.

The author summarizes the AMA's influence in the late 1970s as possibly slipping....but still packs a punch." The article provides specific examples of federal legislation and to what extent the AMA was successful in sponsoring, modifying, or stopping it. Demkovich offers details on the American Medical Political Action Committee (AMPAC) and campaign assistance to specific congressmen. The author additionally addresses other medical associations and portrays them as weak alternatives to the AMA, with the exception of special societies and their unique scientific and technical advancements.

70. Donlan, Thomas G. "AMPAC: It 'PACS' a Punch." *Physicians Management* (November 1986): 65-68.

Donlan's article reviews AMPAC, "The political arm of the AMA." The author looks at the 1986 congressional elections and provides details about how AMPAC selects candidates to support or challenge. Donlan explains how AMPAC and other PACS can legally contribute unlimited funds to a campaign as long as the "independent expenditures" do not breach the insulation between candidate and PAC. The author concludes with AMPACs specific 1986 support to unseat representatives Stark and Jacobs of the House Ways and Means Committee.

71. Felch, William C. "The AMA's Role in Health Legislation. " *American Medical News* (June 22, 1979): 2-4.

This is an excellent, brief article on the process by which AMA policy is established, translated into positions on legislation, presented to the AMA Legislative Council for recommendations to the Board of Trustees, and submitted to Congress or state legislatures as a draft bill or testimonial. The article includes a useful flow chart that clearly explains policy development in the 1970's.

72. Freymann, John Gordon "Leadership in American Medicine." *The New England Journal of Medicine* 270 (1964): 710-719.

The author, as Director of Medical Education at Worcester Memorial, Worcester MA, views American medicine in a negative light and accounts the factors contributing to this condition. Dr. Freymann begins with the contention that AMA is no longer a constructive, well led organization but one that is unimaginative, passive and obstructionist. The author says the years just before WWII were the AMA's "Golden Age" when it was a driving and progressive organization.

Since then, Freymann claims the scientific and academic leaders have left AMA's top positions and gone into specialty societies. He sees a schism between practicing and academic physicians that damages AMA's control of its own destiny. Freymann sees the AMA being dominated now by those concerned about private practice while research and academic physicians are no longer interested in politics. Freymann concludes with a challenge for the AMA to start positively directing change in medicine rather than seeking to stop it. He calls for reform and common effort at all levels.

73. Gray, Charlotte. "AMA Has Five Registered Lobbyists in Washington on Payroll." *CMA Journal* 118 (1978): 1437, 1439, and 1442.

This brief article is an excellent one describing AMA's lobbying process and capability in 1978. The author emphasizes the importance of state medical society participation and the importance of cultivating personal relationships with members of Congress. Gray cites AMA's Washington office statistics of interest, such as 10% of bills introduced into Congress are of relevance to physician practice or that the AMA itself found Congressional sponsorship to introduce 35 pieces of their own legislation in the current Congress. Dr. John Zapp, the Washington Office director, says the AMA lobby serves the interests of all physicians but also helps Congress speed up the legislative process by providing valuable expertise and technical information.

74. Halberstam, Michael J., and Linda B. Halberstam. "Why I'm Finally Joining the AMA." *Medical Economics* 49 (1972): 116-118, 120, 125 and 128.

This article was written during a low point in AMA history, with membership drastically falling and its influence quickly waning. Dr. Halberstam says he refused to join the AMA previously because of its historical fight against national health insurance, Blue Shield and prepaid group health associations. He understands too that specialty societies almost made the AMA obsolete, that other associations like the American Hospital Association and American Public Health Association strongly compete with the AMA, and that the Federal Government now holds the powerful control over medicine once held by the AMA. The Halberstams point out that the AMA is under fire of groups to the right, such as the Congress of County Medical Societies, and left-wing organizations such as Physicians for Social Responsibility. And because of all this, physicians should now join the AMA and strengthen it because they need a strong, overall voice which can bargain in Congress and lobby effectively the legislation conducive to free private practice. The authors then propose specific measures the AMA can do to further strengthen its position (e.g., lobby for periodic re-licensing and re-certification).

75. Hughey, Linda L. "The Resident Voice in Organized Medicine." *Journal of American Medical Association* 241 (1979): 1353-1355.

The author traces the founding, growth, and actions of the AMA's Residents Physicians Section (RPS). Hughey references earlier, short-lived attempts to organize residents since the 1940's. The RPS has strengthened overall AMA membership and benefited the life of residents by giving them a voice in organized medicine, providing them access to malpractice insurance, continuing education and legal assistance. The article includes discussion of state and local resident organizations and the many projects RPS sponsors. When this article was written, one in every six AMA members was either a resident or a medical student. RPS, then, is an important element of organized medicine, introducing the young doctor to political and socioeconomic issues that he or she will have to face in the future.

76. Hyde, Daniel R., P. Wolf, Anne Gross, and Elliott L. Hoffman. "The American Medical Association: Power, Purpose, and Politics in Organized Medicine." *Yale Law Journal* 63 (May 1984): 938-1022.

This 85 page article, with 709 footnotes, is a detailed treatment of the AMA's power in the 1950's and its application towards raising the quality of medical services, determining the conditions of practice and payment, and controlling governmental intervention in health care issues. The article is critical of the AMA in several areas, including previous racial discrimination, disallowing dissident opinions, controlling the nation's supply of doctors, and interfering with national health care program development.

The authors present the AMA as a formidable political lobby which has a primary incentive of protecting individual private physician requests and their fee-for-service system of remuneration.

Details on the AMA's objection with chiropractors, osteopaths, and psychologists as well as compulsory national health insurance are comprehensive, if not totally objective. The extensive footnotes add much more detail and provide a significant bibliography for future study. The authors do credit the AMA for its many important contributions in advancing ethics, medical education, research, product testing, and quality of health care.

The authors address the structure of the association and its linkage with state and local medical societies. They then summarize the sources of AMA social, economic, and political power. The vast majority of the article is dedicated to the application of power, and concludes with recommendations for reform.

77. Keiser, K. Robert, and Woodrow Jones, Jr. "Do the AMA's Campaign Contributions Influence Health Care Legislation?" *Medical Care* 24 (1986): 761-766.

This article posits that AMA political power has been usually overestimated but it does still have a significant impact. The authors show that ideology and party membership have greater influence than AMA contributions. Second, campaign monies have a greater impact over a series of legislative issues than over one key issue. Third, the AMA does have more impact on health policy than does organized labor (AFL-CIO). Fourth, AMA campaign money can influence committee action more readily than general membership of the legislature. Keiser and Jones conclude with the warning, "now that the AMA is clearly exposed as not being invincible, caution should be taken not to underestimate its power."

78. Kosterlitz, Julie. "Organized Medicine's United Front In Washington Is Showing More Cracks." *National Journal* (January 11, 1986): 82-86.

Kosterlitz claims that many factors have led to an increasingly fragmented organized medicine. The author says the AMA prefers to resist any changes which might lessen its power or the quality of patient care. Recent challenges include threats to decrease Medicare payments to doctors, the growth in the number of expensive specialists and their societies. More than 40 medical organizations for example, have offices in Washington. Kosterlitz says actions like AMA's successful battle to stop President Carter's cost containment plan have brought on countermeasures by budget-minded politicians. These congressmen see an erosion of credibility and a failure of organized medicine to regulate itself and voluntarily hold down costs. While the AMA once had unquestioned community support, key groups of citizens like the AARP are at odds with organized medicine over issues like medical cost cuts and who should bear the impact.

79. Lundberg, George D. "The Increasing Representativeness of AMA Leaders." Journal of the American Medical Association. 264(9) (September 5, 1990): 1153-1154.

This brief article provides an excellent summary of the AMA House of Delegates' composition. The author shows how the 436 delegate positions are allocated. Dr. Lundberg maintains the AMA is far more representative now than in its old days when it was "largely the domain of the white, private practice, male physicians." Yet, says the author, the House of Delegates could be restructured to be even more representative of minorities, females, and specialty societies.

80. Pressman, Steve. "Physician's Lobbying Machine Showing Some Signs of Wear." *Congressional Quarterly* (January 7, 1984): 15-19.

This article describes the still powerful, if somewhat lessened, political strength of AMA's lobbying efforts. Pressman cites the association's losing battles with the FTC in 1982 and with Congress in 1983 regarding Medicare payment limitations. The author claims the AMA has been criticized for placing economic health of doctors above the nation's physical health, and has suffered in reputation for its decades of struggle against Medicare. Pressman's article describes the AMA's process for policy development, the role of the American Medical Political Action Committee (AMPAC), and other political competitors in the health care world. Two lengthy sidebars in this article expand upon related topics of the health care lobby.

81. Somerville, Janice. "AMA Scores Legislative Victories on Medicare Issues." *American Medical News* (January 5, 1990): 43.

This brief article shows how successful the AMA political lobby can be during one calendar year. In 1989, association victories were experienced in the basis for Medicare payments to physicians, anti-smoking legislation, right-to-die matters, and self-regulated utilization review programs. Moreover, the Federal Trade Commission cleared the AMA of suspicion of manipulating the supply of physicians and prevent foreign medical graduates from practicing in the U.S.

82. Stacy, James. "How Physicians Fight for Their Point of View." *American Medical News* (June 22, 1979): 4-6.

This article addresses AMA lobbying--past accomplishments, the current process and example issues. Citing AMA Executive Vice President James H. Sammons, the article captures AMA perspectives on the vital necessity to conduct a lobby in an era when over 2,500 health-related bills are considered by each congress. Dr. Sammons says the bills are often poorly thought out and most AMA lobbying "efforts today are directed toward convincing legislators that certain proposals are ill-advised."

83. Wagner, Lynn. "AMA Struggles to Shepherd Diverse Flock." *Modern Healthcare* (July 23, 1990): 34-37.

This is a short article which illustrates the impact that medical specialties have had on fragmenting an organized medicine united under AMA. Wagner begins with interesting statistics on the AMA, e.g., 290,000 members (44% of nation's physicians) and a $200 million annual budget. The author also describes, with praise, the AMA's democratic structure and policy-making process. Wagner then shows how Medicare physician reimbursement reform has led specialty associations like the American College of Surgeons and American College of Radiology to seek their own separate deals with Congress. Wagner says one indication that the AMA's influence may be slipping is the action by Representative Fortney "Pete" Stark to prohibit the AMA from appearing at budget hearings of the House Ways and Means Health Subcommittee. The author concludes, however, that "There's still recognition that the organization (AMA) plays an important role."

84. Wagner, Lynn. "PACs Work Their Influence on The Hill." *Modern Healthcare* (July 9, 1990): 18.

Wagner's article provides an update on the magnitude and activities of healthcare related political action committees (PACs) and some thoughts on their future. The article says there are 259 health-related PACs out of 4,517 PACs in operation. Spending on congressional candidates continues to grow, in spite of their frequent failings to get their friend elected or re-elected to Congress, or their foe defeated by an opponent. PAC advocates claim they help get the right candidate in office, they improve their access to lawmakers, facilitate participation in the political system and reward those who have helped the healthcare interests. Opponents claim PACs are often ineffective, waste money, may cause politicians to be less honest and should be terminated. Some say grass-root members wield the real power and that PACs are not needed. In spite of campaign reform movements since 1974, no major restrictions on PACs are forecasted for the immediate future. Wagner's article includes expenditure figures and strategies by the AMA and AHA.

ORGANIZATION AND MEMBERSHIP

The organization of the AMA consists of a national association with executive officers, Board of Trustees, staff, House of Delegates and various councils. Within the U.S. states and territorial possessions, the association also has 54 state-level groups and the many local societies at county or city level. By the early 1920s, membership in the national association was mandatory to acquire membership in state and local societies. This linkage was furthermore often tied to the state licensing process and the individual hospital credentialing of physicians. Linkage of this nature obviously provided a powerful incentive to join all three levels, thereby immensely strengthening AMA. Today, each individual state society has the authority to link membership requirements, or not, with national. Throughout AMA history, the association has relied on the grass-roots influence and strength of local societies to recruit physicians and organize their efforts towards furthering AMA interests.

Membership at the present time comprises approximately 270,000 physicians who are dues paying members of national AMA. The national association's work, however, generally promotes the interests of most of the over 550,000 physicians in the U.S. As with most organizations, membership will wax and wane with the general economy, and in response to other factors such as dues perceived benefits to members, reputation and focus of the association.

The AMA was still a weak, poorly supported association after its first 50 years of existence. In 1900 for example, the national association had only 8,400 members, or approximately 9% of the nation's physicians. Following the 1901 restructuring and major reforms of the 1900-1910 era, membership jumped to 70,000 (or 50%) in 1910 and 83,000 (or 60%) in 1920.

Over the past thirty years, the AMA has gotten 45 to 75 percent of the nation's doctors to join the national association as full dues paying members. In spite of the major proliferation of medical specialty societies, the AMA remains as the preeminent professional association of physicians.

The following summarizes today's AMA organization, as derived from the *1991 AMA Directory of Officials and Staff.* Like any dynamic association, changes frequently occur in response to mission, functional responsibilities, opportunities, resources and leadership.

1. *Officers.* The association's six officers are comprised of these positions:

--- President
--- President-Elect
--- Immediate Past President
--- Secretary-Treasurer
--- Speaker of the House of Delegates
--- Vice Speaker of the House of Delegates

2. *Board of Trustees.* The board includes a chairman, President, President-Elect and Immediate Past President, as well as several physician members from across the nation. The board includes a medical student trustee and doctor in residency.

3. *The House of Delegates.* This is the policy-making body of the AMA. Proceedings of their actions at annual and interim AMA meetings are documented in yearly *Proceedings of the House of Delegates.* The delegates and alternates are appointed from all U.S. states and territorial possessions, as well as approximately 88 other professional organizations. These others include the U.S. Armed Forces, the Public Health Service, the Veterans Administration, AMA-sponsored special sections (medical schools, medical students, resident physicians, young physicians and hospital medical staff), most major medical specialty associations, academies, colleges, societies and medical insurance associations.

4. *The AMA Staff.* Approximately 1,100 people are employed by the AMA staff. All are under management of the AMA Executive Vice President.

5. *AMA Board of Trustee Councils.*

--- Council on Constitution and Bylaws.
Members include doctors, a lawyer and medical student. This is a fact-finding and advisory committee for constitution and bylaw matters.

--- Council on Ethical and Judicial Matters.

Members include doctors, a lawyer and medical student. This council interprets constitutional and bylaw matters and issues, opinions or ethical concerns. It receives appeals by applicants regarding discrimination, and requests the President appoint investigating juries for ethical issues.

--- Council on Legislation.
Members include doctors, a lawyer, medical student and AMA Auxiliary representative. This council provides surveillance and reviews proposed federal legislation and regulations. It recommends AMA actions on legislative matters and AMA policy.

--- Council on Long-Range Planning and Development.
Members include doctors, a lawyer and medical student. This council studies and makes recommendations on long-range objectives of the association's resources, programs and organization. It anticipates changes in the environment which impact AMA interests.

--- Council on Medical Education.
Members include doctors and a medical student. This council studies and evaluates all aspects of medical education, including the supply of well qualified physicians and the needs of allied health professions. It also functionally manages these committees:

-- Committee on Allied Health Education and Accreditation.

-- Continuing Medical Education Advisory Committee.

-- Graduate Medical Education Advisory Committee.

--- Council on Medical Service.
Members include doctors, a medical student and secretary. This council studies and evaluates social and economic aspects of medical care. It suggests the means for timely development of services. This council also has these committees:

-- Ad Hoc Committee on Peer Review Organizations.

-- Ad Hoc Committee on Rural Health.

--- Council on Scientific Affairs.

Members include doctors, a medical student, Ph.D.s and others. This council advises the AMA on substantial, promising developments in the scientific aspects of medicine and biomedical research that warrant public attention. It advises on professional and public information programs and on opportunities to cooperate with others in joint programs, both domestic and international. The council proposes and evaluates AMA activities involving major scientific projects.

6. *Accreditation Councils, Commissions and Committees.* (AMA provides representatives to these bodies).

--- The Accreditation Council for Continuing Medical Education. Representatives are from the AMA, American Board of Medical Specialties, American Hospital Association, Association for Hospital Medical Education, Association of American Medical Colleges, Council of Medical Specialty Societies and Federation of State Medical Boards of the U.S., Inc.

--- The Accreditation Council for Graduate Medical Education. Representatives are from the AMA, American Board of Medical Specialties, American Hospital Association, Association of American Medical Colleges, Council of Medical Specialty Societies, the Public, the House Staff and the federal government.

--- Joint Commission on Accreditation of Healthcare Organization (JCAHO).

--- Accreditation Program for Ambulatory Health Care of the JCAHO.

--- Accreditation Program for Home Care of the JCAHO.

--- Accreditation Program for Long-term Facilities of the JCAHO.

--- Hospital Accreditation Program of the JCAHO.

7. *Specialty Section Council.* The AMA's bylaws require councils representing the following specialties for the study of scientific, educational and other interests. In addition to AMA

representatives, these councils have members from key specialty colleges, academies, societies, and other associations. There are presently section Councils on:

--- Allergy
--- Anesthesiology
--- Cardiovascular Disease
--- Clinical Pharmacology and therapeutics
--- Colon and Rectal Surgery
--- Dermatology
--- Diseases of the Chest
--- Emergency Medicine
--- Family and General Practice
--- Federal and Military Medicine
--- Gastroenterology
--- General Surgery
--- Internal Medicine
--- Neurological Surgery
--- Neurology
--- Nuclear Medicine
--- Obstetrics and Gynecology
--- Ophthalmology
--- Orthopaedic Surgery
--- Otorhinolaryngology
--- Pathology
--- Pediatrics
--- Physical Medicine and Rehabilitation
--- Plastic Reconstructive and Maxillofacial Surgery
--- Preventive Medicine
--- Psychiatry
--- Radiology
--- Urology

8. *Liaison Committee for Specialty Boards.* This is a large and important committee that has numerous subcommittees dealing with residency, educational and other requirements for the many specialty disciplines.

9. *Other Coalitions, Committees, and Panels.* AMA provides sponsorship and representatives to support these additional areas:
--- AMA National Adolescent Health Coalition.
--- Committee on Medicolegal Problems.
--- Professional Liability Advisory Panel.
--- Informal Steering Committee on Prescription Drug Abuse.
--- The Liaison Committee on Medical Education.

--- Physician Advisory Panel on Radio, Television, and Motion Pictures.

--- Women in Medicine Advisory Panel.

--- AMA Auxiliary. This organization of approximately 75,000 physician spouses is the volunteer arm of the AMA. It raises and distributes money for medical education and research. It sponsors community health programs on a myriad of subjects. The Auxiliary also helps the AMA promote legislation favorable to association interests.

--- The AMA Education and Research Foundation (AMA-ERF). This foundation, managed by the AMA Board of Trustees, funds medical schools, medical research and innovative health care programs. Funding is derived from contributions by medical societies, auxiliaries, physicians, the public and private business.

--- The American Medical Political Action Committee (AMPAC). This committee is the political arm of the AMA with lobbying headquarters in Washington, D.C. AMPAC comprises approximately 50,000 members with state groups across the nation. Individual members include influential grass-roots physicians, spouses and others. The organization fosters political knowledge and political action to advance the interests of the AMA.

Mission, Constitution, Goals and Objectives

The basic mission of the AMA was well documented during its founding in 1847, and has not changed to the present. That mission, stated in article II of the AMA constitution, is "To promote the science and art of medicine and the betterment of public health." The full AMA Constitution follows this section.

In 1984, The Association's House of Delegates reaffirmed four major purposes for which all AMA programming is planned and conducted. These "AMA Purposes" are:

"1. **Representation of the Medical Profession.**--All surveys confirm that representation is the AMA's primary purpose. This function, which must always be consistent with the best interests of the public, is becoming more important than ever before as federal and state governments increase their legislative and regulatory activities.

2. **Provision of Information Related to Medicine.**--This function involves many activities that serve the diverse information needs of the profession and the public. The AMA's role as a leading provider of scientific and socioeconomic information to physicians worldwide is likely to expand as economic and technological forces continue to affect medical practice.

3. **Establishment, Implementation, and Maintenance of Standards of Conduct and Performance.**--The growing diversification of health care delivery will intensify pressures on physicians to uphold the highest standards of professional conduct while providing quality care in a cost-effective manner. The AMA provides guidelines in this area.

4. **Participation in the Establishment, Implementation, and Maintenance of Standards for Medical Education.**--Although the AMA shares this responsibility with other organizations, the Association is a leader in the development of educational policy in medicine and is strengthening its relationships with the academic community.

While these official statements provide good summaries of major AMA focus, it is perhaps difficult to determine the relative importance of these purposes. Moreover, the reader should recognize that mission and priorities have changed to meet the demands within the AMA and those of the external environment. For example, throughout the association's history, promoting the socioeconomic interests of the individual member physician has been at the forefront of the AMA mission. The association's major efforts to isolate "unscientific" practitioners from competing with AMA "scientific" alleopaths is near legendary. Also in the socioeconomic interests of member physicians have been AMA initiatives to: defend doctors' fee-for-services reimbursement and private practice interests from government regulation; promote tort reform and other actions to contain the costs of malpractice insurance; provide, through local societies, group insurance coverage; maximize the flow of scientific and medical information to physicians, as well as promote their basic medical education, residency and continuing education; provide members with advice on medical practice management; improve the image of physicians in the public's eye as a professional with quality health care interests being number one priority; and many other programs to support physician members.

The AMA's mission has also focused on improving the quality of care to individual patients and the public at large. Charges have been made, perhaps deservingly, that AMA ethics serve economic interests, that the association tries to control the number of physicians in order to ensure lucrative practice, and that the AMA has a reactive and defensive political agenda. Nevertheless, the association's activities in the long term have unquestionably benefited the public. Improved ethics, peer review, medical schools, licensing standards, and physician knowledge of drugs, new technologies, diagnostic and treatment processes have all resulted in substantially better capabilities to discover cure and health problems. Moreover, the AMA has helped promote a healthy and safe environment through: evaluating food and drug products; advocating sanitation and public health programs; helping consumer protection agencies alert the public to matters such as hazardous substances and toys; and successfully influence legislation like that requiring seat belts for automobiles.

Constitution of the American Medical Association December, 1990 (Revision)

ARTICLE I--TITLE AND DEFINITION
The name of this organization is the American Medical Association. It is a federacy of its state association.

ARTICLE II--OBJECTS
(*Note:* This is the basic AMA mission which has not changed since 1847.) The objects of the Association are to promote the science and art of medicine and the betterment of public health.

ARTICLE III--STATE ASSOCIATIONS
Constituent or state associations are those recognized medical association of states, commonwealths, territories or insular possessions which are, or which may hereafter be, federated to form the American Medical Association.

ARTICLE IV--COMPONENT SOCIETIES
Component societies are those county or district medical societies contained within the territory of and chartered by the respective state associations.

ARTICLE V--MEMBERS
The American Medical Association is composed of individual members of state associations and others as shall be provided in the Bylaws.

ARTICLE VI--HOUSE OF DELEGATES
The legislative and policy-making body of the Association is the House of Delegates composed of elected representatives and others as provided in the Bylaws. The House of Delegates shall transact all business of the Association not otherwise specifically provided for in this Constitution and Bylaws and shall elect the general officers except as otherwise provided in the Bylaws.

ARTICLE VII--GENERAL OFFICERS
The general officers of the Association shall be a President, President-Elect, Immediate Past President, Secretary-Treasurer, Speaker of the House of Delegates, Vice Speaker of the House of Delegates and fourteen Trustees, including a Resident Physician member and a non-

voting medical student member. Their qualifications and terms of office shall be provided in the Bylaws.

ARTICLE VIII--TRUSTEES

The Board of Trustees is composed of seventeen members, thirteen Trustees elected by the House of Delegates, including a Resident Physician member, a non-voting medical student trustee appointed by the Board of Trustees, and the President, President-Elect and Immediate Past President of the Association. It shall have charge of the property and financial affairs of the Association and shall perform such duties as are prescribed by law governing directors of corporations or as may be prescribed in the Bylaws.

ARTICLE IX--SCIENTIFIC ASSEMBLY

The Scientific Assembly of the American Medical Association is the convocation of its members for the presentation and discussion of subjects pertaining to the science and are of medicine.

ARTICLE X--CONVENTIONS

The House of Delegates shall meet annually and at such other times as deemed necessary or as provided in the Bylaws, in cities or places selected by the Board of Trustees. The Scientific Assembly shall meet at such times as the Board of Trustees deems necessary, or as provided in the Bylaws, in cities or places selected by the Board of Trustees.

ARTICLE XI--FUNDS, DUES AND ASSESSMENTS

Funds may be raised by annual dues or by assessment on the Active Members on recommendation by the Board of Trustees and after approval by the House of Delegates, or in any other manner approved by the Board of Trustees as provided in the Bylaws.

ARTICLE XII--AMENDMENTS

The House of Delegates may amend this constitution at any convention provided the proposed amendment shall have been introduced at the preceding convention and provided two-thirds of the voting members of the House of Delegates registered at the convention at which action is taken, vote in favor of such amendment.

THE HIPPOCRATIC OATH

I swear by Apollo Physician and Asclepius and Hygieia and Panaceia and all the gods and goddesses, making them my witness, that I will fulfill according to my ability and judgment this oath and this covenant:

To hold him who has taught me this art as equal to my parents and to live my life in partnership with him, and if he is in need of money to give him a share of mine, and to regard his offspring as equal to my brothers in male lineage and to teach them this art--if they desire to learn it--without fee and covenant; to give a share of precepts and oral instruction and all the other learning to my sons and to the sons of him who has instructed me and to pupils who have signed the covenant and have taken an oath according to the medical law, but to no one else.

I will apply dietetic measures for the benefit of the sick according to my ability and judgment; I will keep them from harm and injustice.

I will neither give a deadly drug to anybody if asked for it, nor will I make a suggestion to this effect. Similarly I will not give to a woman an abortive remedy. In purity and holiness I will guard my life and my art.

I will not use the knife, not even on sufferers from stone, but will withdraw in favor of such men as are engaged in this work.

Whatever houses I may visit, I will come for the benefit of the sick, remaining free of all intentional injustice, of all mischief and in particular of sexual relations with both female and male persons, be they free or slaves.

What I may see or hear in the course of the treatment or even outside of the treatment in regard to the life of men, which on no account one must spread abroad, I will keep to myself holdings such things shameful to be spoken about.

If I fulfill this oath and do not violate it, may it be granted to me to enjoy life and art, being honored with fame among all men for all time to come; if I transgress it and swear falsely, may the opposite of all this be my lot.

OTHER KEY PROFESSIONAL ASSOCIATIONS

Being the umbrella professional association which represents over 500,000 physicians and the public's healthcare interests, the AMA must work continuously with many other organizations. The followings represent the hundreds of key agencies, societies, and associations, which the AMA often reviews socioeconomic, legal, scientific, and medical policies, programs, plans of action, products, and services. The list is not all inclusive.

American Academy of Neurology (AAN). Established 1948. 2221 University Avenue SE, Station 335, Minneapolis, MN 55414. 10,000 members. Professional society of medical doctors specializing in nerve and nervous system diseases. Maintains placement service. Sponsors research and educational programs. Conducts annual conference. Publishes American Academy of Neurology Membership Directory (annually) and Neurology (monthly).

American Academy of Orthopedic Surgeons (AAOS). Established 1933. 222 S. Prospect Avenue, Park Ridge, IL 60068-4058. 14,500 members. Professional society of orthopedic surgeons certified by the American Board of Orthopedic Surgery to practice orthopedic surgery. Conducts annual meeting. Publishes Bulletin (quarterly).

American Academy of Ophthalmology (AAO). Established 1896. 655 Beach Street, San Francisco, CA 94109. 1,600 members. Supports high-quality eye care and continuing medical education. Monitors legislation affecting ophthalmology and presents to congressional committees and regulatory agencies. Conducts annual conference. Publishes Basic and Clinical Science Course, Ophthalmology (monthly), Directory (biennial) and Argus (monthly).

American Academy of Otolaryngic Allergy (AAOA). Established 1941. 8455 Colesville Road, Station 745, Silver Spring, MD 20910-9998. 1,800 members. Otolaryngologists who are interested in the study, research, and practice of otolaryngic allergy. Offers research fellowship in allergy related to the head and neck. Sponsors scientific meetings and continuing medical education programs. Conducts annual meeting. Publishes AAOA News (quarterly) and Directory (annually).

American Academy of Otolaryngology—Head and Neck Surgery (AAOHNS). Established 1982. 1 Prince Street, Alexandria, VA 22314. 9,000 members. Professional society of medical doctors specializing in otolaryngology and head and neck surgery. Represents otolaryngology in governmental and socioeconomic areas and provides high-quality medical education for otolaryngologists. Coordinates Combined Otolaryngological Spring meetings for six national Otolaryngological societies. Conducts annual meeting. Publishes American Academy of Otolaryngology--Head and Neck Surgery--Bulletin (monthly), Conjoint Directory of the American Academy of Otolaryngology—Head and Neck Surgery (semiannual), and *Otolaryngology—Head and Neck Surgery* (monthly).

American Academy of Pediatrics (AAP). Established 1930. 141 Northwest Point Blvd., PO Box 927, Oak Grove Village, IL 60009-0927. 38,000 members. Sponsors Pediatrics Review and Education Program (PREP). Operates member library of books and journals on pediatric medicine, office practice, and child health care policy. Conducts annual meeting. Publishes AAP News (monthly), Fellowship List (annually), *Pediatrics in Review* (10/year), and other guides and handbooks.

American Academy of Physical Medicine and Rehabilitation (AAPMR). Established 1938. 122 S. Michigan Avenue, Station 1300, Chicago, IL 60603. 3,200 members who are certified as Diplomats of American Board of Physical Medicine and Rehabilitation. Promotes the art and science of medicine and betterment of public health through an understanding and utilization of the functions and procedures of physical medicine and rehabilitation. Sponsors continuing education courses. Conducts annual meeting. Publishes American Academy of Physical Medicine and Rehabilitation--Membership Directory (annually), *Archives of Physical Medicine and Rehabilitation* (monthly), and The Physiatrist (monthly).

American Association of Clinical Urologists (AACU). Established 1969. 800 members. Clinical urologists who are members of the American Urological Association or its sections and the AMA. Its purposes are to stimulate interest in the science and practice of urology and to promote understanding of socioeconomic and political affairs affecting medical practice. Not a referral service for people with urological/medical problems. Conducts annual meeting. Publishes Membership Roster (annually) and Newsletter (bimonthly).

American Association of Electrodiagnostic Medicine (AAEM). Established 1953. 21 2nd Street SW, Station 306, Rochester, MN 55902. 2,531 members. Practicing physicians who are active in electromyography and electrodiagnosis and have made contributions to this field. Objective is to increase and extend knowledge of electromyography and electrodiagnosis and to promote professional and personal association of physicians and surgeons most interested in the field. Conducts annual conventions. Publishes AAEM Case Reports (2-3/year), AAEM Minimonographs (2-3/year), American Association of Electrodiagnostic Medicine--Membership Directory (annually).

American Association of Neurological Surgeons (AANS). Established 1931. 22 S. Washington Street, Station 100, Park Ridge, IL 60068. 3,160 members. Neurological surgeons to promote excellence in neurological surgery and its related sciences. Provides funding for research in the neurosciences. Conducts specialized education. Maintains archives and 300-volume library. Conducts annual meeting. Publishes American Association of Neurological Surgeons Membership Roster (annually), American Association of Neurological Surgeons Newsletter (quarterly), *Journal of Neurosurgery* (monthly), and Neurosurgical Topics (quarterly).

American Association of Pathologists (AAP). Established 1976. 9650 Rockville Pike, Bethesda, MD 20814. 2,000 members. Experimental research pathologists who have made significant contributions to the knowledge of disease. Conducts annual meeting. Publishes AAP Newsletter (quarterly), American Journal of Pathology (monthly), and Membership Directory (annually).

American Association of Plastic Surgeons (AAPS). Established 1921. 10666 N. Torrey Pines Road, La Jolla, CA 92037. Professional society for plastic surgeons with 425 members. Conducts annual scientific program.

American Association of Public Health Physicians (AAPHP). Established 1954. 650 New Town Pike, Lexington, KY 40508. 200 members. Promotes leadership in the field of public health. Speaks for its membership on proposed health legislation at various levels. Conducts educational seminars. Conducts annual meeting. Publishes American Association of Public Health Physicians Bulletin (3/year), Newsletter (annually), and Membership Roster (annually).

American Association for Thoracic Surgery (AATS). Established 1917. 13 Elm Street, PO Box 1565, Manchester, MA 01944. 900

members who are specialists in surgery of the chest region, including cardiovascular surgeons. Encourages investigation and study of intrathoracic physiology, pathology, and therapy. Conducts annual meeting. Publishes *Journal of Thoracic and Cardiovascular Surgery* (annually) and Membership Directory (annually).

American Board of Internal Medicine (ABIM). Established 1936. 3624 Market Street, Philadelphia, PA 19104. Approximately 40 members. Certification board determines qualifications of, administers examinations to, and certify as specialists in internal medicine. Has certified over 91,000 internists and 43,000 subspecialist diplomats and issued 8,600 recertification certificates. Publishes Policies and Procedures (annually).

American Board of Medical Specialties (ABMS). Established 1970. One Rotary Center, Suite 805, Evanston, IL 60201. About 30 members. Acts as spokesman for approved specialty boards. Works with other groups to establish standards, policies and procedures for ensuring continued competence of such physicians. Actively concerned with establishing and maintaining standards for education and qualification for physician specialists' certification procedures. Conducts semiannual meeting. Publishes ABMS Compendium of Certified Medical Specialists--list of over 365,000 board certified specialists (biennial), ABMS Record (periodic), and American Board of Medical Specialties--Annual Report and Reference Handbook (annually).

American Cancer Society (ACS). Established 1913. 1599 Clifton Road NE, Atlanta, GA 30329. 2,500,000 volunteers supporting education and research in cancer prevention, diagnosis, detection, and treatment. Conducts annual meeting. Publishes American Cancer Society--Annual Report, *CA-A Cancer Journal for Clinicians* (bimonthly), *Cancer* (semimonthly), *Cancer News* (3/year), World Smoking and Health (3/year), and Cancer Nursing News (quarterly).

American Chiropractic Association (ACA). Established 1930. 1701 Clarendon Blvd., Arlington, VA 22209. 20,000 members. Promotes the science and art of chiropractic medicine and the public's knowledge of chiropractic medicine. Conducts annual conference. Publishes *Journal of Chiropractic* (monthly), ACA/FYI (monthly), and American Chiropractic Association Membership Directory (annually).

American College of Allergy and Immunology (ACAI). Established 1987. 800 E. Northwest Hwy., Station 1080, Palatine, IL 60067. 3,400 members. Practicing allergists, educators, researchers, and clinical immunologists united to encourage the study, improve the practice, and advance the cause of clinical immunology and allergy. Promotes highest standards. Maintains special program for allergy assistants such as nurses and technologists. Conducts annual congress. Publishes *Annals of Allergy* (13/year), Immunology and Allergy Practice (monthly), Newsletter (bimonthly), and Membership Directory (triennial).

American College of Cardiology (ACC). Established 1949. 9111 Old Georgetown Road, Bethesda, MD 20814. 18,000 members. Professional society of 18,000 physicians, surgeons, and scientists specializing in cardiology and cardiovascular diseases. Operates Heart House Learning Center and library of 1,500 volumes. Conducts annual scientific session. Publishes Accel (monthly), Affiliates in Training (quarterly), *Journal of the American College of Cardiology* (14/year), and Cardiology (monthly).

American College of Chest Physicians (ACCP). Established 1935. 330 Dundee Road, Northbrook, IL 60062. 14,000 members. Professional society of physicians and surgeons specializing in diseases of the chest. Promotes undergraduate and postgraduate medical education and research in the field. Sponsors seminars and forums. Conducts annual scientific assembly. Publishes American College of Chest Physicians Membership Directory (annually), Cardiopulmonary News and Interviews (quarterly), and Bulletin (quarterly).

American College of Emergency Physicians (ACEP). Established 1968. PO Box 619911, Dallas, TX 75261-9911. 13,633 members. Physicians who devote a significant portion of their professional time to emergency medicine. Aim is to provide a unifying direction of purpose in the field, which is a new medical specialty. Encourages training of emergency physicians, with the aim of improving emergency department care in hospitals; conducts continuing education programs for emergency physicians and other healthcare personnel. Conducts annual scientific assembly. Publishes ACEP News (monthly), *Annals of Emergency Medicine* (monthly), and *Foresight* (quarterly).

American College of Gastroenterology (ACG). Established 1932. 4222 King Street, Alexandria, VA 22302. 2,800 members. Professional society of physicians and surgeons specializing in diseases and disorders of the gastrointestinal tract and accessory organs of digestion, including disorders due to nutrition. Conducts annual conference. Publishes *American Journal of Gastroenterology* (monthly).

American College of Healthcare Executives (ACHE). Established 1933. 840 N. Lake Shore Drive, Suite 1130W, Chicago, IL 60611. 23,000 members. Professional society for hospital and health service administrators. Works to: keep members abreast of current and future trends, issues, and developments; shape productive and effective organizational strategies and professional performance; increase the visibility and recognition of the healthcare management profession; act as advocate for health care management in legislative activities and with government agencies; develop cooperation among professional societies and other health care associations in dealing with current issues; strengthen and encourage the profession's code of ethics. Holds educational seminars and training programs on health care management. Conducts annual meeting in conjunction with American Hospital Association and holds annual Congress on Administration. Publishes Directory (biennial), *Frontiers of Health Services Management* (quarterly), *Health Service Research* (bimonthly), *Healthcare Executive* (bimonthly), *Hospital and Health Services Administration* (bimonthly), *Medical Care Review* (quarterly), and Career Mart (career listings).

American College of Legal Medicine (ACLM). Established 1955. 5700 Old Orchard Road, Skokie, IL 60077-1024. 850 members. Persons who hold degrees in medicine and law. To promote and advance the field of legal medicine or medical jurisprudence; arrange for meetings with medical, legal, and professional groups and legislative, judicial, and enforcement bodies interested in any province where law and medicine are contiguous; make available postgraduate training in legal medicine and/or medical jurisprudence. Conducts annual professional clinical conference. Publishes American College of Legal Medicine - Newsletter (periodic).

American College of Nuclear Medicine (ACNM). Established 1972. PO Box 5887, Columbus, GA 31906. 500 members. Physicians and medical scientists in nuclear medicine united to: advance the science of nuclear medicine; improve its benefits to patients; study the socioeconomic aspects of the practice of nuclear medicine; encourage improved and continuing education for practitioners in this and allied fields. Conducts annual scientific program. Publishes ACNM Directory (biennial) and ACNM Report (bimonthly).

American College of Nuclear Physicians (ACNP). Established 1974. 1101 Connecticut Avenue NW, Station 700, Washington, DC 20036. 1,200 members. Nuclear medicine physicians, scientists, and corporations. Objectives are: to foster the highest standards of nuclear medicine service and consultation to the public, hospitals, and referring physicians; to advance the science of nuclear medicine and improve nuclear medicine consultation and service through study, education, and improvement of the socioeconomic aspects of the practice of nuclear medicine; to promote the continuing competence of practitioners of nuclear medicine. Conducts educational seminars and continuing education program. Conducts annual meeting and scientific session. Publishes Directory (annually) and Scanner (10/year).

American College of Obstetricians and Gynecologists (ACOG). Established 1951. 409 12th Street SW, Washington, DC 20024. 29,000 members. Physicians specializing in childbirth and the diseases of women. Sponsors continuing professional development program. Conducts annual meeting. Publishes Bulletin (periodic), Directory of Fellows (biennial), Newsletter (monthly), and Obstetrics and Gynecology (monthly).

American College of Occupational Medicine (ACOM). Established 1988. 55 W. Seegers Road, Arlington Heights, IL 60005. 5,200 members. Physicians specializing in occupational medicine. Promotes maintenance and improvement of the health of industrial workers; works to increase awareness of occupational medicine as a medical specialty. Conducts annual conference. Publishes *American College of Occupational Medicine*--Membership Directory (annually), ACOM Report (10/year), and *Journal of Occupational Medicine* (monthly).

American College of Optometric Physicians (ACOP). Established 1978. 500 members. Optometric physicians and students of optometric medicine. To promote education, research, and total clinical patient care in the field of optometry. Sponsors semiannual continuing education program. Operates the American Board of Optometric Medicine which recognizes achievement within the college and certifies fellowships. Conducts semiannual conference and symposium. Publishes American Journal of Optometric Medicine (quarterly).

American College of Physician Executives (ACPE). Established 1978. 4890 W. Kennedy Blvd., Station 200, Tampa, FL 33609. 4,500 members. Physicians whose primary professional responsibility is the management of health care organizations. Provides for continuing education and certification of the physician executive; the advancement and recognition of the physician executive and the profession. Offers specialized career planning, counseling, recruitment and placement services, and research and information data on physician managers. Conducts annual conference and institute. Publishes American College of Physician Executives-Membership Directory (annually), College

Digest (bimonthly), *Physician Executive: Journal of Management* (bimonthly), and *The Vantage Report* (quarterly).

American College of Physicians (ACP). Established 1915. Independence Mall West, 6th Street at Race, Philadelphia, PA 19106. 63,000 members. Professional society of medical doctors specializing in internal medicine and closely related specialties such as dermatology, neurology, psychiatry, cardiology, gastroenterology, and public health. Sponsors annual postgraduate courses for practicing physicians. Conducts annual scientific meeting. Publishes Annals of Internal Medicine (bimonthly), Directory (periodic), Medical Knowledge Self-Assessment (triennial), and Observer (monthly).

American College of Preventive Medicine (ACPM). Established 1954. 1015 15th Street NW, Station 403, Washington, DC 20005. 2,400 members. Professional society of medical doctors specializing in preventive medicine, public health, aerospace medicine, and occupational medicine. Conducts annual meeting. Publishes ACPM News (quarterly), *American Journal of Preventive Medicine* (bimonthly), Directory of Residency Programs (periodic), Katharine Boucot Sturgis Lectureship (annually), Membership Roster (periodic), and Careers in Preventive Medicine.

American College of Radiology (ACR). Established 1923. 1891 Preston White Drive, Reston, VA 22091. 20,000 members. Physicians and radiologic physicists who specialize in the use of x-ray, ultrasound, nuclear medicine magnetic resonance, and other imaging modalities for the diagnosis of disease and treatment of cancer. Conducts research programs. Offers specialized education and placement services; provides insurance.

American College of Rheumatology (ACR). Established 1934. 17 Executive Park Drive NE, Station 480, Atlanta, GA 30329. 4,700 members. Physicians, scientists, and academicians with a common interest in patients with joint and connective tissue diseases. Encourages study and research, training, and teaching of practicing physicians in care of patients, and development of community facilities for treatment, care, rehabilitation of arthritis patients. Conducts annual scientific meeting. Publishes ACR Membership Directory (annually), ACR Scientific Program (annually), Arthritis and Rheumatism (monthly), Index of Rheumatology (annually), and Landmark Advances in Rheumatology, Dictionary of Rheumatic Diseases, Handbook of Rehabilitative Rheumatology.

American College of Surgeons (ACS). Established 1913. 55 E. Erie Street, Chicago, IL 60611. 50,000 members (fellows). Worldwide organization of surgeons whose working to elevate the standards of surgical education and practice. Sponsors CME and self-assessment for surgeons. Conducts nationwide programs to improve emergency medical services. Conducts annual clinical congress. Publishes American College of Surgeons Yearbook (triennial), *Bulletin of the American College of Surgeons* (monthly), Surgical Forum (annually), Surgery, Gynecology, and Obstetrics (monthly), and Factbook (annually).

American Dental Association (ADA). Established 1859. 211 E. Chicago Avenue, Chicago, IL 60611. 140,000 members. Professional society of dentists concerned with the improvement of the public health and to promote the art and science of dentistry. Inspects and accredits dental schools and other related schools. Produces most of the dental health education material. Compiles statistics on personnel, practice, and dental care needs and attitudes. Conducts research programs at ADA Health Foundation Research Institute. Maintains biographical records of U.S. dentists (past and present). Formerly National Dental Association. Conducts annual meeting. Publishes Accepted Dental Therapeutics (biennial), American Dental Directory (annually), Dental Abstracts (monthly), Dentist's Desk Reference: Materials, Instruments, and Equipment (triennial), Index to Dental Literature (quarterly), News (biweekly), Special Care in Dentistry: Managing Special Patients, Settings, and Situations (bimonthly).

American Gastroenterological Association (AGA). Established 1897. 6900 Grove Road, Thorofare, NJ 08086. 6,400 members. Physicians of internal medicine certified in gastroenterology; radiologists, pathologists, surgeons, and physiologists with special interest and competency in gastroenterology. To study normal and abnormal conditions of the digestive organs and problems connected with their metabolism; to conduct scientific research; to offer placement services. Conducts annual meeting. Publishes AGA Membership Roster (annually), AGA News (quarterly), Gastroenterology (monthly), and Viewpoints on Digestive Diseases (5/year).

American Geriatrics Society (AGS). Established 1942. 770 Lexington Avenue, Station 400, New York, NY 10021. 6,022 members. Professional society of physicians and other health care professionals interested in problems of the aged. Encourages and promotes the study of geriatrics; stresses the importance of medical research in the field of aging. Conducts annual conference. Publishes AGS Newsletter (bimonthly), Directory of Fellowship Programs in

Geriatric Medicine (every 18-24 months), Journal of the American Geriatrics Society (monthly), and Geriatrics Review Syllabus: A core Curriculum in Geriatric Medicine (brochure).

American Group Practice Association (AGPA). Established 1949. 1422 Duke Street, Alexandria, VA 22314. 300 members. Private group practice medical and dental clinics representing more than 21,000 physicians. Compiles statistics on group practice. Sponsors research, patient education, and insurance programs. Provides consulting services and speakers' bureau. Conducts annual conference and congressional forum. Publishes American Group Practice Association--Executive News Service (22/year), Executive News Service (biweekly), Directory (annually), *Group Practice Journal* (bimonthly), and books on administration and operation of clinics.

American Health Care Association (AHCA). Established 1949. 1201 L Street NW, Washington, DC 20005. 9,800 members. Federation of state associations of long-term health care facilities. Promotes standards for professionals in long-term health care delivery and quality care for patients and residents in a safe environment. Focuses on issues of availability, quality, affordability, and fair payment. Conducts seminars that provide continuing education for nursing home personnel. Maintains liaison with governmental agencies, Congress, and professional associations. Conducts annual conference. Publishes AHCA Notes (biweekly), Provider: For Long Term Care Professionals (monthly), A Consumer's Guide to Long Term Care, Thinking About a Nursing Home?, and Welcome to Our Nursing Home.

American Health Planning Association (AHPA). Established 1970. Rhode Island Department of Health, Room 408, Providence, RI 02908. State and local health planning agencies and affiliated organizations and individuals. Conducts research; disseminates information; serves as clearinghouse for health planning activities and concepts; sponsors programs of technical assistance; provides continuing education; maintains speakers' bureau. Conducts 3 conferences/year. Publishes Directory of State and Local Health Planning Agencies (periodic), and TODAY in Health Planning (periodic).

American Heart Association (AHA). Established 1924. 7320 Greenville Avenue, Dallas, TX 75231. 200,000 members. Supports research, education, and community service programs with the objective of reducing premature death and disability from cardiovascular diseases and stroke. Coordinates the fight against heart and circulatory disease. Conducts annual scientific session. Publishes

Arteriosclerosis and Thrombosis: *A Journal of Vascular Biology* (bimonthly), *Cardiovascular Nursing* (bimonthly), *Circulation* (monthly), *Circulation Research* (monthly), Current Concepts of Cerebrovascular Disease and Stroke (bimonthly), *Hypertension* (monthly), Modern Concepts of Cardiovascular Disease (monthly), and *Stroke--A Journal of Cerebral Circulation* (monthly).

American Hospital Association (AHA). Established 1898. 840 N. Lake Shore Drive, Chicago, IL 60611. 45,000 members. Individuals and health care institutions including hospitals, health care systems, and pre- and post-acute health care delivery organizations. Is dedicated to promoting the welfare of the public through its leadership and assistance to its members in the provision of better health services for all people. Carries out research and education projects in such areas as health care administration, hospital economics, and community relations; represents hospitals in a national legislation; offers programs for institutional effectiveness review, technology assessment, and hospital administrative services to hospitals conducts educational programs furthering the in-service education of hospital personnel. Conducts annual meeting. Publishes AHA News (weekly), Guide to the Health Care Field (annually), Hospital Statistics (annually), and *Hospitals* (biweekly).

American Laryngological, Rhinological, and Otological Society (ALROS). Established 1985. PO Box 155, East Greenville, PA 18041. 750 members. Professional society of medical specialists dealing with the ear, nose, and throat. Conducts annual scientific session. Publishes American Laryngological, Rhinological, and Otological Society--Transactions (annually).

American Managed Care and Review Association (AMCRA). Established 1971. 1227 25th Street NW, No. 610, Washington, DC 20037. 450 members. Medical organizations from the managed health care industry representing over 250,000 practicing physicians. Seeks to provide better medical care and to render the most appropriate and economical setting for its delivery. Conducts educational sessions and seminars. Maintains placement service. Conducts annual meeting. Publishes AMCRA Newsletter (10/year), HMO Directory (annually), PPO Directory: And the Industry Report on PPO Development (semiannual).

American Medical Association (AMA). Established 1847. 515 N. State Street, Chicago, IL 60610. 271,000 members. Makes its members aware of significant medical and health legislation. Helps set standards for medical schools, hospitals, continuing medical education, and residency programs. Physician placement service. Represents the medical profession before Congress. Conducts semiannual meeting. Publishes *Journal of the American Medical Association* (JAMA) (weekly), *American Medical News* (weekly), *American Journal of Diseases of Children* (monthly), and monthly Archives for various specialties.

American Medical Association Auxiliary (AMAA). Established 1922. 75,000 members. Physicians' spouses. Raises money for the AMA Education and Research Fund. Sponsors health programs--child abuse prevention, AIDS education, suicide prevention, drug abuse deterrence, prenatal and postnatal care, proper nutrition, and venereal disease awareness. Works with the AMA for sound health legislation. Conducts annual meeting. Publishes Direct Line Newsletter (bimonthly). *Horizons* Newsletter (bimonthly), and Facets Magazine (bimonthly).

American Medical Association - Education and Research Foundation (AMA-ERF). Established 1962. 535 N. Dearborn Street, Chicago, IL 60610. Does not have a membership. Managed by the members of the AMA's Board of Trustees. Receives and distributes funds to support medical education in medical schools in the U.S. and medical research and health care pilot programs.

American Medical Peer Review Association (AMPRA). Established 1973. 810 First Street NE, Station 410, Washington, DC 20002. 1,000 members. Institutions and individuals. Purpose is to develop communications programs for physicians, institutions, and others interested in peer review organizations (PROs). Provides a national forum for the interchange of ideas, techniques, and information relating to medical quality assessment. Conducts courses and on-site assistance programs on increasing physicians' involvement and leadership in PROs, improving practice patterns through review, understanding and using PRO data to improve service delivery, preadmission review, profile analysis, retrospective review, and organizational development. Sponsors placement service. Conducts annual meeting. Publishes AMPRA Bulletin (periodic), AMPRA Review (quarterly), Impact Report (annually), Membership Directory (annually), and Tapes of Annual Session Programs.

American Medical Political Action Committee (AMPAC). Established 1961. 1101 Vermont Avenue NW, Washington, DC 20005. 50,000 members. Interested in political action and increasing its members' political knowledge and awareness. Publishes *Political Stethoscope* (periodic).

American Medical Record Association (AMRA). Established 1928. 919 N. Michigan Avenue, Chicago, IL 60611. 30,000 members. Registered record administrators; accredited record technicians with expertise in health information management, biostatistics, classification systems, and systems analysis. Sponsors Independent Study Program in Medical Record Technology. Conducts annual qualification examinations to credential medical record personnel as Registered Record Administrators (RRA) and Accredited Record Technicians (ART). Conducts annual meeting. Publishes American Medical Record Association--Membership Roster (semiannual), From the Couch: Official Newsletter of the Mental Health Record Section of the American Medical Record Association (quarterly), The Gavel: AMRA State Presidents' Newsletter (quarterly), Journal of AMRA: America's Health Information Leaders (monthly), *Medical Record Educator* (quarterly), QA Section Connection (bimonthly), and *Spectrum* (quarterly).

American Medical Student Association (AMSA). Established 1950. 1890 Preston White Drive, Reston, VA 22091. 25,000 members. Medical students; local, state, and national organizations; premedical students, interns and residents. Seeks to improve medical education by making it relevant to today's needs and by making the process by which physicians are trained more humanistic. Serves as a mechanism through which students may actively participate in the fields of community health through various student health programs. Addresses political issues relating to the nation's health care delivery system and other medical and health issues. Offers specialized education and placement service; conducts research; operates speakers' bureau. Sponsors regional workshops. Maintains 18 task forces and standing committees which publish newsletters, organize educational workshops, and initiate special projects. Conducts annual meeting. Publishes The New Physician (monthly).

American Medical Technologists (AMT). Established 1939. 710 Higgins Road, Park Ridge, IL 60068. 16,500 members. The national professional registry for medical laboratory technologists, technicians, and medical assistants. Bestows various excellence awards and sponsors AMT Institute for Education. Conducts annual conference. Publishes AMT Events and Continuing Education Supplement (8/year) and Manual of the Accrediting Bureau of Health Education Schools.

American Medical Women's Association (AMWA). Established 1915. 801 N. Fairfax Street, Suite 400, Alexandria, VA 22314. 11,000 members. For women holding a M.D. or D.O. degree (approved by medical colleges), women interns, residents, and medical students. Directs its attention to problems facing women in medicine such as career advancement and the integration of professional and family responsibilities. Provides student members with educational loans and personal counseling. Conducts annual meeting. Publishes Journal (bimonthly), Quarterly Newsletter, What's Happening in AMWA (semiannual).

American Nurses' Association (ANA). Established 1896. 2420 Pershing Road, Kansas City, MO 64108. 200,000 members. Member associations representing registered nurses. Sponsors American Nurses' Foundation (for research), American Academy of Nursing, Center for Ethics and Human Rights, International Nursing Center, and American Nurses Credentialing Center. Conducts biennial meeting. Publishes *American Journal of Nursing* (monthly), *The American Nurse* (10/year), Annual Report, Facts About Nursing (semiannual), and Proceedings of the House of Delegates (annual).

American Occupational Therapy Association (AOTA). Established 1917. 1383 Piccard Drive, Suite 301, Rockville, MD 20850-4375. 42,000 members. Registered occupational therapists and certified occupational therapy assistants. Focuses on the active involvement of the patient in specially designed therapeutic tasks and activities to improve function, performance capacity, and the ability to cope with demands of daily living. Conducts research program and compiles statistics. Supports the American Occupational Therapy Foundation, which administers a program of professional training and development in research and provides research information related to occupational therapy. Conducts annual meeting. Publishes *American Journal of Occupational Therapy* (monthly), Developmental Disabilities Specialty Section Newsletter (quarterly), Physical Disabilities Special Interest Section Newsletter (quarterly), and Sensory Integration Special Interest Section Newsletter (quarterly).

American Ophthalmological Society (AOS). Established 1864. Duke University Eye Center, Durham, NC 27710. 225 members. Professional honorary society of physicians specializing in the functions and treatment of the eye. Conducts annual meeting. Publishes *Transactions of the American Ophthalmological Society* (annually).

American Optometric Association (AOA). Established 1898. 243 N. Lindbergh Blvd., St. Louis, MO 63141. 28,000 members. Professional society of optometrists, students of optometry, and paraoptometric assistants and technicians. Purposes are: to improve the quality, availability, and accessibility of eye and vision care; to represent the optometric profession; to help members conduct their practices; to promote the highest standards of patient care. Monitors and promotes legislation concerning the scope of optometric practice, alternate health care delivery systems, health care cost containment, Medicare, and other issues relevant to eye/vision care. Operates Vision U.S.A. program, which provides free eye care to the working poor. Conducts specialized education program; operates placement service. Conducts annual congress. Publishes *American Optometric Association* News (semimonthly), *Journal of the American Optometric Association* (monthly), and *Optometric Economics* (monthly).

American Orthopedic Association (AOA). Established 1887. 222 S. Prospect Avenue, Park Ridge, IL 60068. 300 members. Professional society of bone and joint surgeons. Seeks to further knowledge in the diagnosis and treatment of crippling diseases. Conducts annual meeting. Publishes American Orthopedic Association--Newsletter (3/year) and *Journal on Bone and Joint Surgery* (8/year).

American Osteopathic Association (AOA). Established 1897. 142 E. Ontario Street, Chicago, IL 60611. 18,768 members. Assists in elevating high standards of medical education in osteopathic colleges. CME program for members. Inspects and accredits hospitals and colleges. Conducts board certification program. Sponsors research activities and national examination board. Conducts annual meeting. Publishes American Osteopathic Yearbook, Directory, The D. O. (monthly), and Journal of AOA (monthly).

American Pediatric Surgical Association (APSA). Established 1970. 236 W. Badillo, Covina, CA 91723-1906. About 500 members. Pediatric surgeons certified by the American Board of Surgery. Seeks to provide competent medical care for children. Forum for discussion of ethics involving child care. Presents new concepts and advances in surgical care of infants and children. Conducts annual meeting. Publishes Annual Program Booklet, APSA Membership Directory (annually), Business Meeting Minutes (annually), Cancer Newsletter (annually), and the *Journal of Pediatric Surgery* (monthly).

American Pharmaceutical Association (APhA). Established 1852. 2215 Constitution Avenue NW, Washington, DC 20037. 40,000 members. Works to assure drug product quality, rational drug therapy, and professional education and training of pharmacists. Conducts annual conference. Publishes *American Pharmacy* (monthly), *Pharmacy Today* (weekly), *Journal of Pharmaceutical Sciences* (monthly), The Pharmacy Student (quarterly), Pharmaceutical Directory (annually) and Handbook of Nonprescription Drugs, and Pharmacy Practice (quarterly).

American Physical Therapy Association (APTA). Established 1921. 1111 N. Fairfax Street, Alexandria, VA 22314. 50,000 members. Accredits educational programs in physical therapy. Provides consultation services to physical therapy schools and facilities offering physical therapy services. Conducts annual meeting. Publishes American Physical Therapy Association Progress Report (periodic), *Clinical Management in Physical Therapy* (bimonthly), *Physical Therapy* (monthly), and PT Bulletin (weekly).

American Professional Practice Association (APPA). Established 1959. 292 Madison Avenue, New York, NY 10017. 70,000 members. Provides physicians with various benefits and services such as group insurance and purchase discounts, equipment and automobile leasing, loan plans, investments, and travel programs. Conducts annual economic and tax saving seminar. Publishes *APPA Digest* (bimonthly) and Pension Update (quarterly).

American Psychiatric Association (APA). Established 1844. 1400 K Street NW, Washington, DC 20005. 36,000 members. Further the study of the nature, treatment, and prevention of mental disorders. Concerned with psychiatric education and research; assists in formulating programs to meet mental health needs. Conducts annual convention. Publishes *American Journal of Psychiatry* (monthly), Psychiatric News (semimonthly), *Hospital and Community Psychiatry* (monthly), and Membership Directory (biennial).

American Public Health Association (APHA). Established 1872. 1015 15th Street NW, Washington, DC 20005. 31,500 members. Physicians, nurses, social workers, pharmacists, health administrators, podiatrists, dentists, and other community and mental health specialists. Concerned with environmental, personal, and mental health and public health research; establishes uniform practices and procedures; sponsors job placement services; presents public health awards. Conducts annual conference. Publishes Salubritas (quarterly), and *American Journal of Public Health* (monthly).

American Roentgen Ray Society (ARRS). Established 1900. 1891 Preston White Drive, Reston, VA 22091. 5,200 members. Specialists in diagnostic and/or therapeutic roentgenology. Conducts regional and educational programs; sponsors competitions. Conducts annual scientific meeting with symposium, courses, and exhibits. Publishes *American Journal of Roentgenology* (monthly) and Membership Directory (annually).

American Society of Abdominal Surgery (ASAS). Established 1959. 675 Main Street, Melrose, MA 02176. 9,300 members. Medical doctors specializing in abdominal surgery. Sponsors extensive program of surgical education including study courses, postgraduate programs, lectures, and demonstrations. Conducts three clinical congresses/year. Publishes *Abdominal Surgery* (monthly), and *The Surgeon* (bimonthly).

American Society of Addiction Medicine (ASAM). Established 1954. 12 W. 21st Street, 8th Floor, New York, NY 10010. 3,500 members. Physicians with special interest and experience in the field of alcoholism and other drug dependencies and who wish to share this experience with other professionals in order to extend their knowledge of addictive diseases; promote dissemination of that knowledge; enlighten the public regarding these problems; advance education and research in the field of addiction. Conducts annual medical/scientific conference. Publishes Newsletter (bimonthly).

Association of Schools of Allied Health Professions (ASAHP). Established 1967. 1101 Connecticut Avenue NW, Suite 700, Washington, DC 20036. 1,200 members. Involved in advancement of allied health education, research, and delivery. Assists in communication among schools of allied health professions. Sponsors short-termed programs for allied health education and administration. Liaison to other health organizations and professional groups. Conducts annual meeting and periodic conference. Publishes Allied Health Trends (monthly), Directory (annual), and *Journal of Allied Health* (quarterly).

American Society of Anesthesiologists (ASA). Established 1905. 515 Busse Hwy., Park Ridge, IL 60068-3189. 27,000 members. Professional society of physicians specializing or interested in anesthesiology. Seeks "to develop and further the specialty of anesthesiology for the general elevation of the standards of medical practice." Encourages education, research, and scientific progress in anesthesiology. Conducts refresher courses and other postgraduate educational activities. Maintains placement service and library. Conducts annual meeting. Publishes *Anesthesiology* (monthly), ASA Newsletter (monthly), and Directory of Members (annually).

American Society of Cataract and Refractive Surgery (ASCRS). Established 1974. 3702 Pender Drive, Station 250, Fairfax, VA 22030. 4,500 members. Ophthalmologists interested in anterior segment surgery and refractive corneal surgery. Offers continuing medical education to ophthalmologists on cataract and refractive surgery techniques, intraocular lens designs, and related research areas; assists allied health care professionals in ophthalmology on medical and surgical care of pseudophakic (lens implant) patients. Works to improve public education in the field of eye care. Conducts research in ocular pathology in cataract and refractive surgery. Conducts annual meeting. Publishes ASCRS Roster (biennial), *Journal of Cataract and Refractive Surgery* (bimonthly), and Newsletter (monthly).

American Society of Clinical Pathologists (ASCP). Established 1922. 2100 W. Harrison, Chicago, IL 60612. 45,000 members. Professional society of clinical pathologists, clinical scientists, chemists, microbiologists, and medical technologists. Promotes a wider application of pathology and laboratory medicine to the diagnosis and treatment of disease. Conducts educational programs in clinical and anatomic pathology and laboratory medicine. Conducts semiannual meeting in conjunction with the College of American Pathologists. Publishes *American Journal of Clinical Pathology* (monthly), Family Directory (annually), Laboratory Medicine (monthly), and Newsletter (monthly).

American Society for Clinical Pharmacology and Therapeutics (ASCPT). Established 1900. 1718 Gallagher Road, Norristown, PA 19401-2800. 2,000 members. "To promote and advance the science of human pharmacology and therapeutics and in so doing to maintain the highest standards of research, education, and exchange of scientific information." Provides a Medical Education Program of Continuing Education for practicing physicians. Conducts annual meeting with symposia. Publishes *Clinical Pharmacology and Therapeutics* (monthly).

American Society of Colon and Rectal Surgeons (ASCRS). Established 1899. 800 E. Northwest Hwy., Station 1080, Palatine, IL 60067. 1,500 members. Professional society of surgeons specializing in the diagnosis and treatment of diseases of the colon, rectum, and anus. Offers placement service; conducts research programs. Conducts annual meeting. Publishes *Diseases of the Colon and Rectum*(monthly).

American Society of Cytology (ASC). Established 1951. 1015 Chestnut Street, Station 1518, Philadelphia, PA 19107. 3,600 members. Cytologists, pathologists, and clinicians with M.D.'s; nonmedical professional personnel (Ph.D.'s); associate members are cytotechnologists. Seeks to make the cytological method of early cancer detection universally available to potential victims. Promotes establishment of additional educational and training facilities; encourages implementation of research programs; inspects and accredits cytology laboratories; assists in preparation of national registry examination for cytotechnologists. Conducts annual conference. Publishes *Acta Cytological* (bimonthly) and *The Cytotechnologist's Bulletin* (bimonthly).

American Society for Gastrointestinal Endoscopy (ASGE). Established 1941. 13 Elm Street, PO Box 1565, Manchester, MA 01944. 4,000 members. Gastroenterologists, internists, and surgeons who perform gastroscopic, esophagoscopic, coloscopic and peritoneoscopic examinations. To further the knowledge of digestive disease by endoscopic methods. Conducts annual meeting. Publishes *Gastrointestinal Endoscopy* (bimonthly).

American Society of Hematology (ASH). Established 1957. 6900 Grove Road, Thorofare, NJ 08086. 4,200 members. Hematologists and other persons holding doctorate degrees with an interest in the field. Promotes exchange of information and ideas related to blood and blood-forming tissues and investigation of hematologic problems. Conducts annual meeting. Publishes *Blood* (monthly), Directory of Members (periodically), and Meeting Program (annually).

American Society of Hospital Pharmacists (ASHP). Established 1942. 4630 Montgomery Avenue, Bethesda, MD 20814. 23,000 members. Placement service for its members. Conducts education programs. Sponsors professional liability program. Conducts annual conference and midyear clinical meeting. Publishes American Journal of Hospital Pharmacy (monthly), ASHP Drug Information (annually), ASHP Newsletter (monthly), *Clinical Pharmacy* (monthly), International Pharmaceutical, Handbook on Injectable Drugs (biennial), and Drug Products Information File.

American Society of Internal Medicine (ASIM). Established 1956. 1101 Vermont Avenue NW, Station 500, Washington, DC 20005-3457. 25,000 members. Professional society of physicians specializing in internal medicine. Is concerned with the social, economic, and political factors affecting the delivery of high-quality care. Focuses on the delivery and financing of medical care in areas including access to care, appropriate reform of American health care system, medical and public education, issues affecting the elderly, private and public sector, health insurance and reimbursement, managed care, documentation of physician performance, and medical technology and computerization. Conducts annual meeting. Publishes Contracting and Negotiations Update (bimonthly), *The Internist: Health Policy in Practice* (10/year), *Internist's Intercom* (monthly), and Directory (biennial).

American Society of Maxillofacial Surgeons (ASMS). Established 1947. 120 Oakbrook Center Mall, Oak Brook, IL 60521. 200 members. Professional society of doctors of medicine and doctors of dental surgery who have at least five years of recognized graduate training and experience in maxillofacial surgery and improve and elevate the standard of practice. Conducts annual meeting.

American Society of Plastic and Reconstructive Surgeons (ASPRS). Established 1931. 444 E. Algonquin Road, Arlington Heights, IL 60005. 4,000 members. Professional society of plastic surgeons. Promotes optimal care for plastic surgery patients through research, service, and education activities. Sponsors public/patient education program, clinical symposia, and professional development workshops. Acts as a liaison between members and government and medical organizations. Conducts annual scientific meeting. Publishes American Society of Plastic and Reconstructive Surgeons Combined Roster (annually), *Journal of Plastic and Reconstructive Surgery* (monthly), and *Plastic Surgery News* (monthly).

American Society for Therapeutic Radiology and Oncology (ASTRO). Established 1955. 1101 Market, 14th Floor, Philadelphia, PA 19107. 3,116 members. Physicians who limit their practice to radiation therapy; associate members are scientists who have a major interest "in furthering the aims of the society"; junior members are residents who have completed one year of training in radiation therapy. Aim is "to extend the benefits of radiation therapy to patients with cancer or other disorders, to advance its scientific basis, and to provide for the education and professional fellowship of its members." Conducts annual conference. Publishes ASTRO Membership Directory (annually), ASTRO Newsletter (periodic), and The International *Journal of Radiation Oncology, Biology, and Physics* (periodic).

American Surgical Association (ASA). Established 1880. 136 Vurnett-Womack, Box CB 7245, University of North Carolina at Chapel Hill, Chapel Hill, NC 27599-7245. 780 members. Doctors of medicine. Promotes the improvement of the science and art of surgery.

Conducts annual scientific meeting. Publishes *Annals of Surgery* (monthly) and *Transactions* (annually).

American Thoracic Society (ATS). Established 1905. 1740 Broadway, New York, NY 10019-4374. 9,000 members. Specialists in pulmonary diseases, physicians in the public health field concerned with tuberculosis control, thoracic surgeons, and research workers in lung diseases. Acts as adviser in scientific matters. Conducts annual conference. Publishes American Journal of Respiratory Cell and Molecular Biology (monthly), *American Review of Respiratory Disease* (monthly), ATS News (bimonthly), and Membership Roster (biennial).

American Urological Association (AUA). Established 1902. 1120 N. Charles Street, Baltimore, MD 21201. 6,100 members. Professional society of physicians specializing in urology. Conducts annual scientific meeting. Publishes AUA Today (monthly), *Journal of Urology* (monthly), and Membership Roster (biennial).

Association for the Advancement of Health Education (AAHE). Established 1937. 1900 Association Drive, Reston, VA 22091. Almost 10,000 members. Purpose is concern with advancement of health education and achievement of good health for all Americans. Conducts annual meeting. Publishes Health Education (monthly) and Directory of Institutions Offering Specialization in Health Education (biennial).

Association of American Medical Colleges (AAMC). Established 1876. One Dupont Circle NW, Washington, DC 20036. Over 2,200 members including medical schools, teaching hospitals, academic medical societies, and graduate affiliate medical colleges interested in the advancement of medical education, health care and research. Develops and administers the Medical College Admissions Test (MCAT) and the Medical Science Knowledge Profile test (MSKP). Conducts annual meeting. Publishes Weekly Report, Academic Medicine (monthly), Curriculum Directory (annually), Directory of American Medical Education (annually), and Medical School Admission Requirements (annually).

Association of American Physicians and Surgeons (AAPS). Established 1943. 9203 Lake Braddock Drive, Burke, VA 22015. Represents physicians in medical economics, public relations and legislation. Conducts an expert witness program. Conducts annual meeting. Publishes AAPS News (monthly), Emergency Bulletin (periodic), and Legal Consultation Service.

Association for Hospital Medical Education (AHME). Established 1954. 1101 Connecticut Avenue NW, Station 700, Washington, DC 20036. 600 members. Physician directors of medical education in hospitals and clinics and other health profession educators. Conducts educational programs and workshops for members and others in the area of graduate and continuing medical education. Conducts annual institute. Publishes Membership Directory (annually), Newsletter (monthly), and AHME Congressional Record.

Association of Life Insurance Medical Directors of America (ALIMDA). Established 1889. 1 Monarch Pl., Springfield, MA 01133. 800 members. Professional society of medical directors of life insurance companies. Conducts annual scientific meeting. Publishes Association of Life Insurance Medical Directors of America--Transactions (annually) and *Journal of Insurance Medicine* (quarterly).

Association of Military Surgeons of the U.S. (AMSUS). Established 1891. 9320 Old Georgetown Road, Bethesda, MD 20814. Physicians, dentists, veterinarians, nurses, pharmacists, dietitians, therapists, and others of commissioned and/or equivalent in the Army, Navy, Air Force, Public Health Service, and Veterans Administration; Reserve and National Guard officers are also eligible for membership. Advances all phases of federal medicine and allied sciences related to federal health services. Conducts annual meeting. Publishes *Military Medicine* (monthly).

Association of University Radiologists (AUR). Established 1953. 1891 Preston White Drive, Reston, VA 22091. 1,200 members. Physician and non-physician scientists who have been appointed to a university faculty. Seeks to: encourage excellence in laboratory and clinical investigation, teaching, and clinical practice; stimulate interest in academic radiology as a medical career; advance radiology as a medical science; provides a forum for university-based radiologists to present and discuss results of research, teaching, and administrative issues.

Auxiliary to the National Medical Association (ANMA). Established 1935. 1012 Tenth Street NW, Washington, DC 20001. Composed of spouses of active members of the National Medical Association (NMA); widows and widowers of former members. Purposes are to: create a greater interest in the NMA; assist and encourage the medical profession in its efforts to educate and serve the public in matters of sanitation and health; develop and promote a national program on health and education with subcategories in community needs, legislation, and human relations. Conducts workshops on teenage pregnancy, breast self-examinations, high blood pressure screening, and sickle cell anemia screening. Plans and implements an annual youth forum under the auspices of the March of Dimes Birth Defects Foundation. Provides youth with professional guidance and the opportunity for peer exchange in the areas of mental and physical health; deals with the health of newborns, health services, nutrition, and teenage pregnancy. Also conducts programs for youth on parenting, socially transmitted diseases, nutrition, birth defects, and continued education after pregnancy. Conducts annual meeting. Publishes Membership Directory (periodic), Newsletter (quarterly), and book of standard procedures.

Blue Cross and Blue Shield Association (BCBSA). Established 1982. 676 N. Clair Street, Chicago, IL 60611. To promote the betterment of public health and security; to secure the widest public acceptance of voluntary nonprofit, prepayment of health services; to provide national services to local Blue Cross and Blue Shield Plans. Contracts with federal government as administrative agency for federal health programs; sponsors and conducts programs on health care and prepayment issues. Publishes Inquiry: The *Journal of Health Care Organization, Provision, and Financing* (quarterly).

Congress of County Medical Societies (CCMS). Established 1966. PO Box 12489, Oklahoma City, OK 73157. Increases communications among county medical associations. Publishes *Private Practice* (monthly).

Contact Lens Association of Ophthalmologists (CLAO). Established 1962. 523 Decatur Street, Station 1, New Orleans, LA 70130-1027. 2,000 members. Active and resident ophthalmologists and doctors of osteopathy specializing in ophthalmology. Objective is to disseminate scientific information on ophthalmology. Provides for the sharing of techniques and expertise; make available statistics and information on related courses, seminars, meetings, and special events. Conducts annual conference. Publishes CLAO Directory (biennial), *CLAO Journal* (quarterly), CLAOfile (quarterly), and CLAOgram (monthly).

Council of Medical Specialty Societies (CMSS). Established 1965. PO Box 70, Lake Forest, IL 60045. 24 members representing almost 300,000 physicians. Works to improve the quality of health care in the United States and to promote excellence in physician education. Promotes communication among medical specialty organizations. Concerned with patient safety programs and with medical education. Forum for discussion and policy-making by medical specialties societies on issues affecting medical practice. Conducts three meetings per year. Publishes Executive Report (monthly).

Federation of American Health Systems (FAHS). Established 1966. 1405 N. Pierce, No. 311, Little Rock, AR 72207. 1,000 members. Privately- or investor-owned (for-profit) hospitals. Presents President's Achievement Award and Individual of the Year Award. Maintains speakers' bureau. Compiles statistics on the investor owned hospital industry. Conducts annual meeting. Publishes Annual Report, Directory of Investor-Owned Hospitals, Hospital Management Companies, and Health Systems (annually), FAHS Review (bimonthly), Federation of American Health Systems Hotline (biweekly), and State-to-State Report (periodic).

Federation of State Medical Boards of the United States (FSMB). Established 1912. 2630 W. Freeway, Suite 138, Ft. Worth, TX 76102-7199. 65 members. State medical examining and licensing boards (including nine osteopathic boards). Conducts annual meeting. Publishes Federation Bulletin (monthly), FSMB Newsletter (quarterly), Handbook (annually), and Legislative and Regulatory Exchange (annually).

Gastrointestinal Pathology Society (GIPS). Established 1979. Dept. of Pathology, Cleveland Clinic Found, 1 Clinic Center Drive, Cleveland, OH 44195. 145 members. Medical doctors and Ph.D.'s: others with an interest in gastrointestinal pathology. Disseminates information and works to increase knowledge about the pathology of the gastrointestinal tract; encourages the development of gastrointestinal pathology as a specialized field. Conducts annual meeting. Publishes American Journal of Surgical Pathology (monthly), and Gastrointestinal Pathology Society--Newsletter (semiannually).

Group Health Association of America (GHAA). Established 1959. 1129 20th Street NW, Suite 600, Washington, DC 20036. 1,000 members. Group practice prepayment health plans and related organizations that support the Health Maintenance Organization movement. Conducts research programs and specialized education seminars; compiles statistics. Conducts annual institute meeting. Publishes GHAA News (bimonthly), HMO Managers Letter (biweekly), Medical Directors Conference Proceedings (semiannually), Proceedings of Annual Institute.

Health Insurance Association of America (HIAA). Established 1956. 1025 Connecticut Avenue NW, Station 1200, Washington, DC 20036. 340 members. Accident and health insurance firms. To promote development of voluntary insurance against loss of income and financial burdens resulting from accident and sickness. Holds individual insurance forums. Conducts annual meeting. Publishes Bulletin (periodic), Directory (annually), Executive Report (monthly), and Sourcebook of Health Insurance Data (biennial).

International College of Surgeons (ICS). Established 1935. 1516 N. Lake Shore Drive, Chicago, IL 60610. 14,000 members. General surgeons and surgical specialists in 111 countries maintaining official relations with the World Health Organization. Promotes the universal teaching and advancement of surgery and its allied sciences. Maintains library open to researchers, individuals working in the profession, and the public. Organizes postgraduate clinics around the world; conducts lecture series and periodic congresses; offers grants, scholarships, and loans for residencies, research, and advanced study in surgery. Conducts biennial conference. Publishes International College of Surgeons Newsletter (3/year), International Surgery (quarterly), and Membership Directory (every 2-3 years).

Joint Commission on Accreditation of Healthcare Organizations (JCAHO). Established 1951. One Renaissance Blvd., Oakbrook Terrace, IL 60181. Establishes standards and conducts voluntary accreditation programs to healthcare organizations such as hospitals, mental health centers, home care organizations, hospice programs, rehabilitation programs, substance abuse treatment facilities, long-termed care facilities, and various healthcare facilities. Sponsors continuing education programs. Participating are members of the American Medical Association, American College of Physicians, American Dental Association, American College of Surgeons, American Hospital Association, and American Medical Association. Publishes Home Care Bulletin (quarterly), JCAHO Perspectives (bimonthly), *Quality Review* Bulletin: *Journal of Quality Assurance* (monthly), and Plant, Technology, and Safety Management Series (quarterly).

Medical Group Management Association (MGMA). Established 1926. 104 Inverness Terr. E, Englewood, CA 80112. 10,000 members. Persons actively engaged in the business management of medical groups consisting of three or more physicians in medical practice with centralized laboratory, X-ray, medical records, and business functions. Sponsors educational training programs. Provides placement and information services. Compiles statistics. Conducts annual conference. Publishes Administrators' Bookshelf (annually), Cost and Production Survey Report (annually), Health Exchange (quarterly), Medical Group Management Journal (bimonthly), Medical Group Management--

Management Update (11/year). Medical Group Management Washington Report (monthly), MGMA Directory (annually), MGMA Membership Salary and Fringe Benefit Survey Report (annually), and Special Reports and Surveys (annually).

National Association of Employers on Health Care Action (NAEHCA). Established 1976. 240 Crandon Blvd., Suite 110, PO Box 220, Key Biscayne, FL 33149. 100 members. Corporate members who educate and assist business in health care management and delivery and QA. Conducts health care management research. Analyzes federal legislation providing information to congressional committees on health legislation and its effects on health care systems. Conducts annual and regional conferences. Publishes Employer's Guide to Purchasing Managed Health Care Services (periodic), Health Action Letter (monthly), NAEHCA Blue Book Digest of HMOs (annually), and NAEHCA Blue Book Digest of PPOs (annually).

National Medical Association (NMA). Established 1895. 1012 Tenth Street NW, Washington, DC 20001. 14,500 members. Professional society of black physicians. Represents major specialties of medicine. Conducts symposia and workshops. Currently planning to establish a library and a physician placement service. Conducts annual scientific meeting. Publishes Journal of the National Medical Association (monthly), Developmental Disabilities Specialty Section Newsletter (quarterly), Physical Disabilities Special Interest Section Newsletter (quarterly), and Occupational Therapy Week.

Physicians Forum (PF). Established 1939. 220 S. State Street, Chicago, IL 60604. Promotes development of a national health service for all financed by a progressive income tax surcharge. Conducts annual meeting. Publishes Newsletter (quarterly) and Physicians Forum Bulletin (quarterly).

Physicians for Social Responsibility (PSR). Established 1961. 1000 16th Street, Suite 810, Washington, DC 20036. 55,000 members. Educates the public on the medical effects of nuclear war. Educates the public on effects of national policy pertaining to arms control issues. Conducts annual conference. Operates a speaker bureau. Publishes Briefing Papers (periodic), PSR Annual Report and PSR Monitor (bimonthly) and PSR Report (quarterly).

Radiological Society of North America (RSNA). Established 1915. 2021 Spring Road, Station 600, Oak Brook, IL 60521. 24,000 members. Radiologists and scientists in fields closely related to radiology, radium, electricity, and other branches of physics related to medical science. Conducts annual scientific assembly. Publishes Directory of Members (annually), Radiographics (bimonthly), and *Radiology* (monthly). Conducts annual conference. Publishes Investigative Radiology (monthly).

Renal Physicians Association (RPA). Established 1973. 1101 Vermont Avenue NW, Station 500, Washington, DC 20005. Physicians specializing in the treatment of renal (kidney) diseases. Promotes optimal care and high standards of treatment for patients. Serves as a national representative for physicians engaged in the study and management of patients with kidney and related disorders. Provides resources for the development of national policies concerning kidney disease such as ESRD legislative and network activities, federal funding for related research, and studies relative to treatment procedures and common practices. Conducts annual meeting. Publishes RPA News (quarterly) and ESRD Program Legal Resource Manual.

Society for Investigative Dermatology (SID). Established 1937. Dept. of Dermatology, 2074 Abington Road, University Hospitals of Cleveland, Cleveland, OH 44106. 2,300 members. Professional society promoting research in dermatology and allied subjects. Conducts annual conference and quarterly regional meeting. Publishes *Journal of Investigative Dermatology* (monthly).

Society of Medical Consultants to the Armed Forces (SMCAF). Established 1945. 4301 Jones Bridge Road, Bethesda, MD 20814-4799. 1,000 members. Professional society of physicians and surgeons who have been in active military service and who have acted as consultants to the Surgeon General of the Army, Navy, or Air Force. To preserve and encourage the association of civilian consultants and military medical personnel and to assist in the development and maintenance of the highest standards of medical practice in the Armed Forces. Conducts annual conference. Publishes Newsletter (3/year) and Roster (every 2-3 years)

Society of Nuclear Medicine (SNM). Established 1954. 136 Madison Avenue, 8th Floor, New York, NY 10016-6760. 12,200 members. Professional society of physicians, physicists, chemists, radiopharmacists, nuclear medicine technologists, and others interested in nuclear medicine, nuclear magnetic resonance, and the use of radioactive isotopes in clinical practice, research, and teaching. Disseminates information concerning the utilization of nuclear phenomena in the diagnosis and treatment of disease. Offers placement bureau. Conducts annual meeting. Publishes The *Journal of Nuclear*

Medicine (monthly), *Journal of Nuclear Medicine Technology* (quarterly), Newsline (quarterly), and Society of Nuclear Medicine Membership Directory (every 3 years).

Society of Thoracic Surgeons (STS). Established 1964. 401 N. Michigan Avenue, Chicago, IL 60611-4267. 2,817 members. Surgeons who confine their practice to the field of thoracic-cardiovascular surgery. Objectives are: to improve the quality and practice of thoracic and cardiovascular surgery as a specialty; to strengthen and establish basic standards in training programs; to encourage clinical and basic research; to promote the professional development of those surgeons specializing in the field. Conducts annual meeting. Publishes Annals of Thoracic Surgery (monthly).

U.S. Department of Health and Human Services (HHS)
Public Health Service (PHS)

*** National Institutes of Health (NIH).** Its mission is to improve the health of the American people through increased knowledge and understanding of disease. Its focus is medical research funding almost 40% of all biomedical research in the United States such as research grants supporting universities, medical schools, hospitals, and other research institutions. Most of the research money is dispersed to 12 constituent research institutes; the names of each indicating its central focus:

1. National Cancer Institute
2. National Institute on Aging
3. National Institute of Child Health and Human Development
4. National Institute General Medical Sciences
5. National Heart, Lung, and Blood Institute
6. National Institute of Allergy and Infectious Diseases
7. National Institute of Dental Research
8. National Institute of Neurological and Communicative Disorders and Stroke
9. National Institute of Arthritis, Musculoskeletal, and Skin Diseases
10. National Institute of Diabetes, Digestive, and Kidney Diseases
11. National Institute of Environmental Health Services
12. National Eye Institute
13. National Center for Nursing Research

*** Alcohol, Drug Abuse, and Mental Health Administration (ADAMHA).** Principal federal agency addressing the problems of alcohol, drug abuse, and mental illness providing assistance to state and community programs. Conducts research in its own laboratories and through grants to other agencies and programs. Provides annual grants to states for treatment and prevention.

* **Food and Drug Administration (FDA).** Assures the safety of foods, drugs, radiological devices and other biological products involved in interstate commerce. It inspects food processing and drugs (for safety and effectiveness).

* **Centers for Disease Control (CDC).** Concerned with prevention and control of chronic diseases and death from environmental and workplace hazards. Use education to reduce health risks. High priority is prevention and control of AIDS. Assists state with locating causes of infectious and communicable diseases. Trains state and local public health officials.

* **Health Resources and Services Administration (HRSA).** Helps integrate the publicly and privately financed health services programs. Provides technical assistance for updating health care facilities. Provides leadership for the education, training, supply, and quality of the United States health personnel. Assists states and communities in setting up emergency medical services.

* **Health Care Financing Administration (HCFA).** Merger in 1877 of Office of Long-termed Care, the Bureau of Quality Assurance, Medicare, and Medicaid. Concerned with development and enforcement of standards for nursing homes. Administers Medicare, Medicaid, and the End-Stage Renal Disease Program. Publishes Health Care Financing Review (quarterly) and periodic special reports on Medicare and Medicaid.

* **Veterans Administration (VA).** Since 1988 the VA has been a cabinet level department. It provides a wide range of benefits including health services. A total system of care, the VA system currently has 172 hospitals (82,000 beds), 95 nursing homes (9,000 beds), and financial care for over 31,000 veterans in some 3,100 community nursing homes. It also provides outpatient care and a variety of other care including home care. Veterans who have some health problems connected with their service in armed forces are clearly entitled to be cared for within the VA system. If there is space available, veterans with non-service-connected disabilities, who cannot afford private care; those over 65 regardless of disability to pay and also the spouse or child of a totally and permanently disabled veteran; the widow or child of a veteran, who died from a service-connected disability. There are no deductibles or coinsurance charges.

*** Occupational Safety and Health Administration (OSHA).** Established in 1970, OSHA is part of the Department of Labor. The Occupational Safety and Health Act was passed to assure, as far as possible, safe and healthful working conditions for every man and woman in the nation, and also to preserve our human resources. OSHA issues and enforces standards and regulations that govern the work environment and the work practices used. It periodically inspects establishments covered by OSHA legislation. OSHA's role in health affairs will increase as man increases his knowledge of the effects of hazardous substances, practices, and machinery in the workplace.

*** Environmental Protection Agency (EPA).** Established in 1970. It combined 15 environmental control programs from various federal agencies, working with regional, state and local governments. It sets and enforces standards involving the environmental areas of air, water, pollution waste management, pesticides, noise, and radiation. Its efforts are directed toward improving the quality and safety of the environment.

*** Federal Trade Commission (FTC).** Established to protect the public against anti-competitive behavior, unfair and deceptive business practices. In recent years it has moved against what is perceived to be anti competitive forces in the health field. It has moved against the AMA's Code of Ethics because it banned advertising and patient solicitation; also, the AMA's role in the accreditation of medical schools. The FTC does not involve itself in a bona fide professional matter or in matters governed by state law, but it does retain the authority to monitor and take action over business or economic matters.

Part Two

Functional Roles, Key Issues, and Outlook for the Future

6

AMA'S ROLE IN PHYSICIAN SUPPORT AND DEVELOPMENT

This set of readings focuses upon the American Medical Association's relationship with and impact on the physician profession and practice. The development of and impact of the Flexner Report is examined by some, since it facilitated the AMA's rise to primacy within health education. A number of the authors look at AMA's efforts to upgrade (or, more cynically, control) physician education and supply. The controversies regarding physician shortages and surpluses are covered here. Subsequent reform proposals, as encapsulated in such outputs as the Millis Report and the Project in Medical Education at the University of Buffalo, are shown to demonstrate that AMA thinking on medical education has never been static.

Other significant education policy issues that are covered include the controversy over Foreign Medical Graduates (FMGs); efforts to reform the physician credentialing process; the rapid growth of continuing medical education (CME) and the allied health professions; growing concerns over malpractice law; and the shortage of general practitioners. With varying degrees of activity and effectiveness, the AMA has become involved in these and a variety of other areas of concern to physicians, attempting to meet new challenges while preserving traditional physician autonomy and prerogatives.

A number of the authors provide critical commentaries on the results of AMA physician activities. In particular, they argue that the Association has not worked hard enough to diversify medical school enrollments (by increasing the number of nonwhite and female students, among other things). Nor has the AMA encouraged significant ethical training for physicians, in their eyes. These criticisms merge with perceptions of a more general AMA complacency and self-interestedness with respect to the increasing social roles and responsibilities of the physician.

The authors in this section would agree that the AMA has earnestly attempted to serve physician interests. They would differ, however, on whether or not these efforts have been adequate, given the rapidly changing world of American medical care and evolving patient and public needs.

(A) Books

85. American Medical Association. *Council on Medical Education, Future Directions for Medical Education.* Chicago, American Medical Association, 1982.

This report, produced by the American Medical Association's Council for Medical Education and adopted by the AMA House of Delegates on June 15, 1982, represents the AMA's official response to new controversies and challenges in physician training that developed during the seventies and early eighties. The document was over three years in the making, and the product of six AMA task forces and contributions from other medical groups such as the American Academy of Family Physicians, the American Board of Medical Specialties, and the Association of American Medical Colleges.

The thirty-six AMA policy recommendations in the report cover 43 pages of text, divided into ten different sections based upon content area and/or stage of medical education. In addition, there is an equally-long "Historical Survey Appendix to Future Directions for Medical Education", which briefly details a number of events which have affected the direction of American medical education in the nineteenth and twentieth century.

In the first section, the Council declares that "the major theme of this report is the balance between generalism and specialism required to permit individuals to develop into well-educated physicians who possess a broad perspective of society, extensive knowledge of the biomedical sciences, experiences in the several defined areas of clinical medicine, a thorough education in a specialty, and an incentive to continue their professional education throughout their careers" (p. 1). A particular concern running throughout the report is that current medical education overemphasizes specialization at the expense of breadth of knowledge. In the view of the Council, this results in inflexible and overly-narrow analysis of patient problems, and a potential inability "to provide many elements of general care required by most patients" (p. 2).

The following sections of the report suggest how broadly-based training and criteria for judgment can be incorporated into various stages of education. The Council recommends that medical schools consider a wider range of factors in admission decision, and give less weight to standardized test scores. Medical school curricula should also be more frequently revised and evaluated for their provision of diverse forms of knowledge (as opposed to narrowly scientific and clinical training). Additionally, "the first year of postdoctoral medical education for all graduates should consist of a broad year of general training" (p. 23). Specialty boards and state licensing agencies should vigorously preserve and upgrade standards, but only in consultation with medical schools, and the medical profession as a whole. Foreign medical schools must also be examined carefully to determine the rigor and breadth of their programs.

In the report's final section ("The American Medical Association and Medical Education"), the Council declares that given the organization's importance and responsibilities, it must "continue to participate vigorously . . . in all matters related to medical education" (p. 43).

86. American Medical Association. "Section on Medical Schools: The Medical Profession: Enduring Values and New Challenges, "Conference Proceedings, February 25-27, 1987." Chicago, IL: American Medical Association, 1988.

This work is the collected proceedings of a 1987 conference jointly sponsored by the American Medical Association, the Association of American Medical Colleges, and the American Hospital Association. As Ira Singer, AMA Conference Coordinator, says in the Foreword, "the co-sponsors undertook this conference to determine how practicing physicians and medical educators can enhance the desirability of medicine as a career and can continue to attract highly qualified applicants to medical school" (p. v).

The text of the proceedings runs to about 260 pages, and, after the "Remarks of Sponsoring Organizations" and introductions, is divided into four major parts: "The New Physician", "The Changing Medical Profession", "The Public's Perception of Medicine", and "Meeting New Challenges and Changing Responsibilities". In the initial remarks, James H. Sammons of the AMA points out that AMA surveys show some slippage in the public's perceptions of physicians. While some of the negative feelings are due to the scapegoating of physicians for the high cost of health care, "the AMA Council on Ethical and Judicial

Affairs has emphasized we have to reexamine our values, including those of our students, and assess our limitations" (p. 11).

A number of speakers use AMA research data to explore trends in physician income and supply, and the attitudes of doctors and medical students. Most prominent in this respect is Steven V. Seekins, AMA Vice President, Public and Professional Communications, who outlines "AMA Studies on Public Attitudes".

Michael Collins, a founder of the Young Physicians Section within the AMA, discusses "The Outlook of the Young Physician", and suggests that younger doctors are more likely to be female, in greater debt, and more concerned with lifestyle factors in practice than their older counterparts. Roy Schwarz, AMA Assistant Executive Vice President for Medical Education and Science, talks about "the Changing Profession: A Physician's Perspective". He provides a profile of the "typical" physician in 1987, talks about the nature of professionalism, and paints a generally bleak picture regarding how recent changes in medical practice have degraded the professional nature of medicine.

In "Medicine and Professionalism", John K. Iglehart (Special Correspondent of the New England Journal of Medicine) describes AMA attitudes toward the Health Care Quality Improvement Act of 1986: "The AMA was a strong advocate of the peer review protections but it lobbied vigorously against a publicly sponsored clearinghouse on physician data and argued that the locus for this clearinghouse function should be within the private sector and more clearly engage in a partnership between the AMA and the Federation of State Medical Boards" (p. 152).

87. Carnegie Council. *Progress and Problems In Medical and Dental Education.* San Francisco, CA: Jossey-Bass, 1976.

This report by the Carnegie Council addresses some of the problems of health-manpower education narrowing its focus to medical and dental education, such as too much dependence on FMGs, geographic maldistribution of health manpower, and shifting patterns of over specialization of medical education. As congress looks at federal legislation, this report urges "a policy of sustained and consistent federal support of medical and dental education, along with the provision of strong incentives towards needed changes, rather than excessive controls."

In chapter four, the Carnegie Council, preferring a three-year physician education program, strongly recommends acceleration of doctors' medical education. This would reduce the costs of medical education as well as the shortage of physicians. They suggest (1) revising medical education course work to allow completion in three years, (2) medical education to include summer course work, (3) advance standing for students who had "extensive premedical preparation," (4) reducing the number of total years for premedical and medical education combined, and (5) eliminating freestanding internships (which the AMA approved in 1970) and integrating them with first year-residencies.

The book also addresses the fact that physician's assistant (PA) programs are costly because their faculty and equipment requirements were similar to medical education programs. The Carnegie Report agrees with the AMA's view that PA programs should be conducted in close relationship to MD training.

In chapter five, the Council examines the National Health Service Corp. (NHSC) which was established in 1970. The supporters of this legislation felt that in view of the AMA's history of opposition to anything looking like socialized medicine, the chances of enactment were questionable. But their efforts were successful and the AMA has "consistently supported the NHSC, while showing particular support for policies that require periodic review of the need for corps members in any given area."

88. Carter, Richard. *The Doctor Business.* Garden City, NY: Doubleday & Company, Inc., 1961.

In this work, Richard Carter, a medical journalist, provides a generally critical look at the behavior of U.S. physicians in general, and the American Medical Association in particular. The twelve chapters of the book (covering about 250 pages) provide explorations into such topics as "Dollar Doctrine", "Insuring the Doctor", "AMA vs. Government" and "The Customer is Sometimes Right". The author sees the fee-for-service system (defended vigorously by physicians) as the primary source of the problem, declaring it to be "inefficient and uneconomical . . . scientifically obsolescent" (p. 20).

The AMA is portrayed by Mr. Carter as the prime mover and defender of this exploitative system, using "propaganda, lobbying funds, and various forms of coercion to enforce its belief that laissez-faire is essential to good medical treatment" (p. 27). The AMA is also hypocritical, since it is also willing to support and engage in restrictive, anticompetitive behavior to preserve its own power (for example, restricting the supply of physicians). According to the author, the AMA also acts as Big Brother with respect to physicians, monitoring and recording behavior that goes against AMA policies and transmitting it to local medical societies on request.

More positive aspects of AMA activity are briefly mentioned: Association efforts to improve medical school education and restrict "quackery". But the overall balance sheet is clearly negative. AMA efforts have produced a physician shortage. The organization has also (until fairly recently) opposed the very notions of health insurance and group practice, and still lobbies against any effective system of national health insurance, or insurance for the poor and elderly. The AMA resists any moves toward imposing the scrutiny of outsiders on medical practice, and is overly protective toward incompetent physicians. It also opposes any attempts to reduce "unnecessary surgeries". The hostility and fear of the AMA's leadership with respect to any significant reforms in the current system verges on hallucination and paranoia.

With respect to reforming the current system, Mr. Carter expresses some optimism, calling for "socialized medicine" not in the sense of government ownership, but of "medicine that is of optimum use to society" (p. 194). Despite AMA opposition, the author foresees the development of more group practices, and the spreading practice of prepaid care "in an irreversible trend away from fee medicine and toward community control" (p. 254).

89. Ginzberg, Eli. *From Physician Shortage to Patient Shortage.* Boulder, CO: Westview Press, 1986.

Subtitled "The Uncertain Future of Medical Practice", this edited work contains seven essays (written by such eminent health service researchers as Harold S. Luft and Rosemary A. Stevens) addressing the troubled present and uncertain future of physician practice in the United States. Five of the essays are based upon presentations made at the Cornell University Medical College Second Conference on Health Policy, which was held in New York City on February 27-28, 1986. Additional introductory and concluding essays are supplied by the editor, Eli Ginzberg.

M. Roy Schwarz ("Physician Personnel and Physician Practice") examines surveys of public attitudes toward physicians conducted by the American Medical Association, and finds a mixed picture. Until 1985, the AMA surveys revealed a steady decline in the public image of physicians. More recently, "the earlier deterioration . . . has ended and there are strong indications of an upturn. . . . [But] while the overall picture is encouraging, there is still much room for improvement" (p. 45).

With respect to manpower issues, the AMA committed itself in 1981 to market-oriented approaches to solving shortage and surplus problems, while gradually reducing the number of medical graduates.

"In 1975 the AMA House of Delegates accepted the integration of the first post-MD year of graduate medical education with subsequent years. As a result, freestanding internship programs were no longer approved, and the total number of graduate medical education programs decreased" (p. 46). In addition, the AMA favors the end of Medicare funding for alien FMGs, while supporting well-designed medical education exchange programs. AMA-accredited programs also license many badly needed allied health practitioners.

Association studies are also used by Joan B. Trauner et al. ("A Lifestyle Decision: Facing the Reality of Physician Oversupply in the San Francisco Bay Area") to document how the attractiveness of the Bay Area has led to an extreme oversupply of both new and veteran physicians. With the high cost of practice, physicians have had to tradeoff income for lifestyle. A 1983 AMA survey showed that Bay Area physicians were disproportionately likely to be in salaried group practice and HMO positions, with relatively low pay. "Readily evident is the fact that most groups in the San Francisco Bay area offer rates below national averages" (pp. 129-130).

90. Green, Joseph S., Sarina J. Grosswald, Emanuel Suter, and Davis B. Walthall III, Editors. *Continuing Education for the Health Professions*. San Francisco, CA: Jossey-Bass, 1984.

This book on learning theory, adult education, and management principles is designed to help plan and implement continuing education activities, primarily health profession schools. It deals with both theoretical foundations and practical applications.

The book is divided into four parts, part one looks at the theoretical foundations of learning proposed by the authors and the relationship of motivation to the participants of learning. Part one is designed to provide practical applications for increasing health professionals' participation.

Part two deals with "Ways Continuing Education Serves the Health Professions" as the title connotes. A 1981 AMA study reflected that physicians spend almost thirteen days a year for formal CME, plus considerable time in informal and self-directed studies. This section also provides a brief historical review of CME from the early efforts by the AMA (1906) to develop CME activities at the county level (which failed), to reactivation after publication of the Flexner Report in 1911, the AMA establishment of an accreditation program for CME, and various CME studies sponsored by the AMA. The AMA supports the trend of shifting responsibility for CME to the community hospital.

In part three, the authors look at some of the theoretical and practical aspects of continuing education and program development while describing the individual components of educational development, i.e. needs assessment, educational activities design, and evaluation.

Part four looks at strategic management's approach to decision making in continuing education. In its conclusion, it answers several questions raised. It explains how concepts and quality elements were learned earlier and how an organization's continuing education activities can be improved.

91. Hunt, Andrew D. *Medical Education, Accreditation and the Nation's Health.* East Lansing, MI: Michigan State University Press, 1991.

Subtitled "Reflections of an Atypical Dean", this book examines the various interrelationships between medical schools, their relevant professional associations (particularly the American Medical Association), and the accreditation process. Dr. Hunt was founding dean of the medical school at Michigan State University, and is currently a part-time Associate Dean at Mercer University School of Medicine. The text is short (about 150 pages), and divided into six chapters.

In Chapter 2, the author outlines "The AAMC and Its Relationship to the AMA". In a short historical section, he emphasizes how closely the two organizations have been intertwined. Since the improvement of medical education was a major goal of the AMA, it worked closely with the American Association of Medical Colleges (established in 1876) to encourage the application of "the German model" to U.S. medical schools. "The new wave of medical education, espousing science, more stringent entrance requirements, and increased intellectual performance, while clearly necessary, did meld with the larger political, economic, and social goals of the AMA" (p. 21).

Dr. Hunt also points out that the Flexner Report, while having a major policy impact, was evolutionary rather than revolutionary in its findings. The AMA had in fact already completed its own survey of medical education, with findings that would be almost identical to those of Flexner. But the AMA intentionally downplayed its own research and encouraged the Carnegie Foundation to commission its own study. "Some accounts of this relationship credit those discussions with reaching an agreement that a repetition of the AMA inquiry by a foundation would remove any suggestion that the AMA had acted in its own self-interest and confirm that the schools were indeed as they had stated" (p. 29).

The symbiotic relationship between the AMA and the AAMC continued. From 1911 through 1922, the AAMC always held its annual conference in Chicago at the same time as that of the Council on Medical Education and Hospitals of the AMA. In 1942, the Liaison Committee on Medical Education was formed, with equal representation for both organizations. They have continued to work closely together on accreditation matters, as described in Chapter 5 ("Accreditation of Medical Schools").

Currently, the LCME has an expanded membership, including the AMA and AAMC (six representatives each), two public members, two student members, and a Canadian from that nation's accrediting body, the CACMS. There is also a Federal Government presence, with an Office of Education member. Dr. Hunt concludes that "in a sense, the history of medical school accreditation recapitulates that of the AAMC and AMA. . . . The partnership with the AMA in the formation of the LCME . . . consummates the relationship with the establishment of a vitally influential power center" (p. 136).

92. Kletke, Phillip R., William D. Marder, and Anne B. Silberger. *The Demographics of Physician Supply: Trends and Projections.* Chicago, IL: American Medical Association, 1987.

This study, produced by three members of the AMA Center for Health Policy Research, is a short (six chapters and 58 pages) analysis of the changes in physician supply, medical education and clinical practice that have occurred in the Twentieth Century. According to James F. Rodgers, Director of the AMA Center, the most important purpose of this work is "to introduce the AMA Demographic Model of the Physician Population. This model makes it possible to project the size and composition of the physician population under a number of different policy scenarios" (p. ix). The findings therefore have implications for the contemporary political debate over funding for medical education, and the relative supplies of the various physician specialties.

In the first two chapters, the study points out what other studies (such as the 1980 GEMENAC report) have found: that the active physician population, which had declined after the issuance of the Flexner report, expanded sharply beginning in the Sixties. The number of foreign medical graduates (FMGs) went up until 1975, when it leveled off. The physician to population ratio is now the highest of the 20th Century.

But the AMA report goes further, portraying a profession of declining attractiveness. In recent years, U.S. medical school applications have declined even more sharply than acceptances, resulting in a steadily decreasing applicants to acceptance ratio (now at 1.8). The drop would have been even greater had it not been for the growing numbers of female applicants (now 36% of the total). New medical school graduates labor under the burden of an increasingly onerous educational debt burden.

As a consequence of all of this, the composition of the active physician population is significantly changing. On the whole, physicians in 1985 were younger and more female than their 1970 counterparts. Some specialties, such as anesthesiology, internal medicine and pediatrics, grew rapidly, while others, such as family practice and surgery, fell behind. By 1985, physicians were practicing more weeks each year, but seeing fewer patients each week. With respect to earnings, "from 1981 to 1985, real income (in 1981 dollars) for the all-physician category rose from $93,000 to $95,700, a statistically insignificant increase of only 2.9 percent" (p. 31).

In Chapter 5, the report offers projections to the year 2000. These include a continued growth in the physician population (even with stringent controls on FMGs), with more females. With declining medical school enrollments after 1989, the growth of the "surplus" will level off by 2000, but still remain.

In the concluding chapter ("Future Research Directions"), the authors state that "with the development of the demographic model, the AMA has expanded its capabilities to plan and prepare for the future. By preparing its own projections of the physician population, the AMA can base its projections on the most recent data and can incorporate into the model the factors which are most relevant to the medical profession" (p. 57).

93. Knowles, John H., Editor. *Views of Medical Education and Medical Care.* Cambridge, MA: Harvard University Press, 1968.

This slim (169 pages of text) volume contains the transcripts of a series of lectures sponsored by the Lowell Institute and Massachusetts General Hospital in 1966. The seven essays, including the views of clinicians, education administrators, a physicist, and the then-Lieutenant Governor of Massachusetts (Elliot Richardson) provide the reader with some differing perspectives on the challenges facing medical education.

In "The Rationalization of Health Services", John Knowles uses the American Medical Association in a discussion of the "defects of syndicalism and vested interest" (p. 82) in the medical education system. He concludes that the AMA often acts in a self-interested fashion, and that its recommendations are not always in the best interests of medical education as a whole.

94. Lippard, Vernon W. *A Half-Century of American Medical Education: 1920 - 1970.* New York, NY: Josiah Macy, Jr. Foundation, 1974.

Vernon Lippard, a retired physician and medical school faculty member, wrote this concise (twelve chapters and 124 pages) book to provide an accessible, concise history of U.S. medical education development since the general adoption of the Flexner Report's recommendations between 1910 and 1920. The book contains numerous references to American Medical Association efforts in the medical education area.

The author credits the AMA with being a primary force for medical education reform from its founding in 1847 through the Flexner period. The AMA's Council on Medical Education, in alliance with the Association of American Medical Colleges, succeeded in upgrading and tightening state medical education regulations, and driving many low-quality medical schools out of business. Curricula were lengthened and made more science-based.

From 1920 to 1970, medical school education continued to improve. In "Specialization and the Specialty Boards" (Chapter X), Dr. Lippard notes the participation of groups such as the AMA Section of Ophthalmology in the development of rigorous standards for certification of physician specialists. In a similar fashion, the AMA-sponsored Citizens Commission on Graduate Medical Education endorsed certification of family practice physicians in 1966. The author emphasizes the powerful influence of the AMA in the entire movement toward specialization: "The AMA established the requirements for and, after inspection, approved internships; and it joined with the specialty boards in approving residencies and determining the training requirements for board examinations" (p. 95).

In Chapter XI ("National Organizations and Foundations"), Dr. Lippard looks at the darker side of AMA activities. He suggests that, for political reasons, the AMA refused to limit the number of residencies offered by hospitals--which led to many poorly organized and supervised educational experiences. The AMA also failed to vigorously support increased medical school funding in the period after 1945. "In summary, as it [the AMA] became more concerned with protecting the economic interests of practicing physicians it became less progressive in its concern for education" (p. 105).

95. McGuire, Christine H., Richard P. Foley, Alan Gorr, Ronald W. Richards and Associates. *Handbook of Health Professions Education*. San Francisco, CA: Jossey-Bass Publishers, 1983.

This lengthy (543 pages) work contains twenty-five contributions dealing with numerous aspects of health education. In Part One, "Trends and Priorities in Health Professions Education", the major health services fields (such as medicine, nursing, pharmacy, and allied health) are covered. Part Two encompasses "research on health professions education", including significant findings. The final section, Part Three, looks at important socioeconomic factors that are prompting change within health service education programs.

In "Allied Health", by Cecil G. Sheps, the role of the American Medical Association's Committee on Allied Health Education and Accreditation is briefly described. Sheps notes that despite the role of the AMA Committee in designing and implementing accreditation procedures, "many allied health professionals do not support that effort due to the committee's involvement with the AMA" (p. 123). AMA involvement will continue, however, as long as the allied health professions are unable to fund the establishment of a unified independent accrediting body.

Julius B. Richmond and Milton Kotelchuck, in "Political Influences: Rethinking National Health Policy", conclude that major federal government health care interventions of the Sixties (especially Medicare and Medicaid) came about despite rather than because of the attitudes of the health professions. The American Medical Association and other organizations "had abdicated responsibility or were actively resisting proposals that an overwhelming majority of the American people recognized as desirable" (pp. 389-390). At this point, though, the health professions have reconciled themselves to a large federal presence: "even the AMA no longer advocates the abolition of Medicare" (p. 396).

96. Miller, George E. *Educating Medical Teachers*. Cambridge, MA: Harvard University Press, 1980.

This book is primarily an account of innovations in medical education during the Fifties and Sixties. In particular, it recounts the beginning of reform efforts through the Project in Medical Education at the University of Buffalo. The author writes as a significant participant in these efforts as a faculty member at the University of Buffalo and the University of Illinois. But the book is certainly not an autobiographical account; equal attention is devoted to numerous other reform educators.

The American Medical Association is briefly discussed in Chapter 9 ("Assimilation and Integration"). According to Miller, the AMA "has eased into the turbulent waters of educational research and development on only a few occasions, but they were important events if short-lived" (p. 198). He mentions the 1961 Joint Study Committee of the AMA and AAMC that produced the report "Lifetime Learning for Physicians", as well as the AMA medical education fellowships offered between 1969 and 1974 at the University of Illinois Center for Educational Development. An AMA-CED Physician Self-Assessment Study (a byproduct of the fellowship program, conducted between 1972 and 1974) is also described. According to Miller, "the AMA Division of Education has maintained an interest in documenting and encouraging further work on this vital element of sound individualized continuing education" (p. 200).

97. Millis, John S. *A Rational Public Policy for Medical Education and its Financing.* New York, NY: National Fund for Medical Education, 1971.

Popularly known as "the Millis report", this work, commissioned by the National Fund for Medical Education, had significant impact on thinking concerning national medical education policy in the 1970s. Its policy recommendations-- expanded medical school enrollment, greater student diversity, and the establishment of a Commission on Medical Education, among others--are presented in eight concise (158 pages) chapters.

The author acknowledges the current role of the American Medical Association (through the Joint Liaison Committee of the Association of American Medical Colleges and the AMA's Council on Medical Education) in setting medical education standards. Throughout the text, he relies on AMA research data to draw conclusions, and frequently quotes AMA officials to support his conclusions. Dr. Millis refers approvingly to the AMA House of Delegates decision to phase out freestanding internships by 1975. However, he also declares that existing accreditation (which centrally involves the AMA) is a "roadblock to change" (p. 73).

The Millis recommendations for change would keep the AMA as a central participant in medical education policy, since physician members of his proposed Commission on Medical Education would be selected by the AMA, along with the specialty societies. In the concluding chapter, the author stresses that the Commission should be established as soon as possible, given the urgent tasks it will face.

98. Millman, Michael L. *Politics and the Expanding Physician Supply*. Montclair, NJ: Allanheld, Osmun & Co., Publishers, Inc., 1980.

This book describes the relationships between the federal government, state governments, and medical institutions and interest groups that affect the level of medical school enrollment (and thus the number of physicians) in the United States. The author is a research associate with the Conservation of Human Resources Project at Columbia University. His purpose here is to show how the lack of state and federal government communication and coordination, and the direct dealings between the federal government and medical institutions (what the author terms "private federalism") during the Sixties and Seventies, led to wasteful and ineffective planning--and an unexpected physician surplus in the Eighties and beyond.

Based upon the author's doctoral dissertation, the book is short (153 text pages) and divided into eight chapters. In "The Medical Education Sector" (Chapter 2), the historical influence of the American Medical Association over medical education is outlined. The Liaison Committee on Medical Education, an official accrediting agency for medical schools (recognized by the U.S. Office of Education) has six AMA Council on Medical Education representatives. Similarly, AMA personnel sit on the residency review committees for graduate medical education used by the Liaison Committee on Graduate Medical Education. The AMA also has considerable leverage (through state medical societies) over the state licensure process. Until the Seventies, many believed that the AMA was using its influence to restrict medical school enrollments.

The AMA was successful in its efforts to prevent direct federal support for medical education through the Fifties. In fact, the Association established its own loan program, but the required interest payments were rather high. "By 1963, the AMA position had become one of support for construction [of medical schools] and public neutrality--tempered with last-minute, behind-the-scenes opposition--on the question of student loans" (p. 25). The Health Professions Education Assistance Act of 1963 was significantly modified in response to AMA criticism. However, the AMA continued to warn against the dangers of overdependence upon the federal government for any type of aid, and proposed amendments to the Administrative Procedure Act to protect medical schools from "excessive" federal involvement. By the late Sixties, "the constrictionist policies of national and local organized medicine has given way . . . to an advocacy on behalf of increasing the physician supply, a change culminating in the joint AMA-AAMC policy statement of 1968" (p. 104). Additional medical schools were established, and enrollments rose sharply. The nation concentrated on producing more doctors, only to find a decade later that it might wind up with far too many.

99. Mullan, Fitzhugh. *White Coat, Clenched Fist.* New York, NY: Macmillan Publishing Company, Inc., 1976.

This book, subtitled "The Political Education of an American Physician", is an autobiographical account of the author's experiences in the 1960s civil rights and peace movements, medical school and practice that heightened his consciousness and disapproval of inequities within U.S. society in general, and its health care system in particular. The book's eleven chapters, with titles such as "Seize the Hospital to Serve the People", attest to Dr. Mullan's growing discontent and radicalization.

On the whole, Dr. Mullan feels that the AMA is a force for reaction in health care. "To many of us the American Medical Association symbolized medicine in America. Overfed and complacent, the 'voice' of organized medicine seemed completely self-serving and ignorant of the health problems that beset many Americans. . . . On issue after issue the AMA supported the rich, the entrenched, and the reactionary" (p. 50). The Student American Medical Association (SAMA) is portrayed as an irrelevant and ineffective organization that fails to provide meaningful experiences for its members. The author concludes by expressing his hope that younger physicians will turn away from conventional, organized medicine and the AMA, and work for the interests of all the people, not just the rich or influential.

100. Percell, Elizabeth F., Editor. *Recent Trends in Medical Education.* New York, NY: Josiah Macy, Jr. Foundation, 1976.

This work contains the edited presentations given by a number of medical education scholars at a Macy Foundation conference in Aspen, Colorado in September 1975. The purpose of the conference was to "consider innovations taking place in the schools and future directions of education at all levels--from premedical studies through postgraduate medical training" (p. vii). The nineteen presentations span about 280 pages of text covering topics such as "the admission process", "independent study programs", "a new paradigm for medical education", "problems in evaluation and examination", and "medical education 1985: a forecast".

The essay by William D. Holden ("Development in Graduate Medical Education") is in part devoted to the efforts undertaken since the mid-Fifties by such groups as the American Medical Association to meet the national challenge of producing an adequate supply of family practice physicians. After studying the problem with the Association of Medical Colleges and the American Academy of General Practice, the AMA's Council on Medical Education approved the establishment of two-year residencies in general practice. By 1973, however, the number of AMA-approved residencies had fallen from 258 to 51, while the number of general practitioners had dropped to 53,946 (14.7% of all physicians).

However, there has been growing interest in the family practice specialty; which was proposed by the AMA in a 1966 Council report. According to Holden, "the rapid growth of this specialty appears to be the result of a recognition by graduating students of the concept of a family practitioner as a personal physician to his patients, in contrast to the organ and systems-oriented practice characteristic of most specialists" (p. 255). In 1975, the Coordinating Council on Medical Education (which includes the AMA among its parent bodies) published a report calling on medical schools to encourage their students to go into the primary care area, including the development of residencies. However, Holden cautions that "the future will be determined by the academic stature of the specialty in university medical centers, and the professional satisfactions of daily practice (p. 256).

Another essay, "The Medical Student, 1975", by Davis G. Johnson, points out that while the caliber of the average entering medical student has risen sharply, this has had one unfortunate byproduct: a significantly more stressful, competitive academic environment. However, a humanizing counter trend has begun to change this. One example of this is "the new student advocacy system of the American Medical Student Association (AMSA) formerly the Student American Medical Association (SAMA) which seeks to help protect student rights at the institutional level" (p. 47). The AMSA also is helping to develop model primary care curricula and lobbying medical schools to adopt such programs. Promoting an increase in the enrollment of minorities in health professions schools is another goal of the AMSA.

101. Raffel, Marshall W., and Norma K. Raffel. *The U.S. Health System*, Third Edition. New York, NY: John Wiley & Sons, 1989.

This is a concise (eleven chapters and 322 text pages) and widely-used comprehensive text on the development and functioning of the U.S. health care system. Within it, the authors cover the impact that the American Medical Association has had, particularly with respect to medical education and practice.

In Chapter 1 ("History of Medical Education and Medical Practice in America"), Raffel and Raffel provide a detailed description of the origins of the AMA, and the obstacles it faced in its medical education reform efforts in the nineteenth century. The chapter also outlines the progress that was made at the turn of the century, particularly with the formation of the AMA Council on Medical Education, and its reform alliance with the AAMC. The breakthrough that took place with the Flexner Report significantly enhanced AMA power, and it gained official control over medical education (in alliance with other groups) with the establishment of the Liaison Committee on Medical Education in 1942. However, the simultaneous rise of specialty societies within medicine would reduce the extent of AMA control over physicians.

The remainder of the chapter discusses the relationships between the AMA and educational developments such as postgraduate school, internships, the Millis Commission, and specialty boards. The authors also describe what they feel are more negative and anticompetitive aspects of AMA behavior (opposition to group practice, for example).

Most other references to the AMA can be found in Chapters 4 and 5, "Medical Practice" and "Nurses and Other Health Professionals". In "Medical Practice", the authors allude to the AMA's efforts to increase physician fees, and its denials that physicians are in fact unfairly profiting from their patients (the target income hypothesis). Raffel and Raffel conclude that the AMA "probably truly does represent the views of its members" (p. 92). The strength of the AMA through its structure of state and local societies is explored. However, "the AMA, though still influential, has become less able to resist the many changes that are being made in medical practice" (p. 96).

In "Nurses and Other Health Professionals", the interactions that the AMA has had with chiropractors, nurses, physician assistants and allied health personnel are briefly mentioned. AMA opposition to chiropractors, once quite intense, has been weakened by time and successful litigation by chiropractors against restrictive practices. The AMA has attempted to reduce physician-nurse tensions, in conjunction with the American Nurses Association, through the National Joint Practice Commission. The Association has expressed concerns about the expansion of physician assistants, fearing a future decrease in the demand for physician services and fees.

102. Rothstein, William G. *American Medical Schools and the Practice of Medicine*. New York, NY: Oxford University Press, 1987.

This fairly lengthy (335 pages) and detailed book is a combined history and policy analysis of American medical education from 1750 to the present. The author, a professor at the University of Maryland, Baltimore Campus, has divided the presentation into five time periods: 1750 - 1825, 1825 - 1860, 1860 - 1900, 1900 - 1950, and after 1950. In each time period, he looks at the state of medical science and medical care, the structure of medical training, and the various social groups that were influential in the establishment of the prevailing medical practices of the period.

Until the Nineteenth Century, medical education was largely by apprenticeship. Beginning in the early 1900s, however, medical schools became a more important medium for physician training, replacing the apprenticeship system. In fact, "the American Medical Association was organized in 1847 largely as a reaction to the increased number of physicians educated by the medical schools" (p. 63). These doctors established medical societies, and called for restrictions on medical school enrollment. But the medical schools themselves preferred larger numbers of students.

AMA members also wanted higher quality medical education, and attempted to apply more advanced educational principles as they populated many of the better medical schools in the late 1800s. Many AMA presidents spent some time on medical school faculties. In the 1900 - 1920 period, the Association vigorously advocated the development of internship programs and residency systems for more realistic education.

In 1905, the AMA established its Council on Medical Education as an information clearinghouse. It also established standards for medical schools. The following year, the Association conducted a comprehensive inspection of all medical schools, using its own standards for evaluation. To bolster its case for reform, the AMA persuaded the Carnegie Foundation to undertake its own study of medical schools (though, to enhance the apparent credibility and objectivity of the study, it wanted its own involvement to remain secret).

The Carnegie Foundation's chosen investigator, Abraham Flexner, used the AMA standards in his research. The report became legendary for its alleged impact on American medical education reform, but Dr. Rothstein argues that medical school modernization would probably have occurred anyway, and the Flexner Report ultimately served the cause of academic elitism.

The AMA Council on Medical Education conducted several other surveys between 1911 and World War II. In general, the reports concluded that medical education was improving, but lower enrollments were still needed. When this recommendation met with public disapproval, the AMA modified its stance, with the House of Delegates calling for an expansion of the best schools.

After World War II, the chief issue in medical education became a perceived national shortage of physicians. The AMA initially opposed virtually all proposals for federal government subsidization of physician training or medical school construction. By the early Sixties, however, it had modified its stance on government funds for school construction, and formally endorsed federal aid for medical school operations in 1968.

In the Seventies, AMA concerns with medical education centered around reforming internship and residency programs. In 1970, the AMA called for the elimination of rotating internships. According to Dr. Rothstein, this has adversely affected physician education. As a response, "the AMA Council on Medical Education, in a repudiation of the 1970 AMA policy, recommended in 1982 that the 'first year of postdoctoral medical education for all graduates should consist of a broad year of general training'" (p. 318).

103. Schofield, J. R. *New and Expanded Medical School, Mid-Century to the 1980s*. San Francisco, CA: Jossey-Bass, 1984.

Schofield divides this work into four parts. Part one, Medical Schools and the Supply of Physicians, describes how the United States went from a surplus of physicians about the beginning of the twentieth century to a shortage by the middle of the century. He goes on to relate some of the methods used to relieve the shortage, with expanding existing medical schools and creating new ones. Organized in 1949 by supporters from all walks of life (including the AMA), the National Fund for Medical Education provided financial support for medical schools. In the late 1950s the AMA began to contribute funds directly to the medical schools while opposing legislation that would provide direct funding to the schools -- especially if it was involved with any kind of compulsory health insurance. This attitude changed, however, in 1968 when Congress, with full endorsement of the AMA, passed Federal Legislation authorizing construction funding and modified matching funds provisions for medical schools.

Part two, Medical School Administration, looks at the roles and functions of medical school deans and their staffs. Chapter Five deals with the founding of the new medical school in areas such as planning the facilities, acquiring the staff (teaching and ancillary), funding the programs, and erecting activities and programs.

In Part three, the author addresses the resources necessary for a medical school: 1) Financial resources - Where do they come from? How are they spent? 2) Student and Faculty Facilities - Where to build? What size? 3) The Medical Library and its capabilities, and 4) Teaching the hospital's characteristics and parts.

In Part four, Schofield describes the components of a physician's medical education and how it evolved to where it is today. Some of the problems faced and recommendations for improving such programs are also provided.

104. Yaggy, Duncan and Patricia Hodgson, Editors. *How Many Doctors Do We Need?* Durham, NC: Duke University Press, 1986.

This short (approximately 160 pages) work is based on the 1985 Tenth Private Sector Conference. The conference was supported by the American Medical Association, the Duke University Medical Center, and the Duke Endowment. It "focused on two questions: Is there a surplus of physicians now, or in prospect? If there is, what should be done about it, if anything?" (p. ix).

One of the conference participants, John A. D. Cooper (President, Association of American Medical Colleges) points out that while most discussion focuses on the need to reduce a physician surplus, there is still great need for additional doctors in some parts of the U.S. There is therefore some merit to an expansive medical school enrollment policy. "In 1968 the Association of American Medical Colleges and the American Medical Association adopted a policy which said that a place should be provided for every qualified student who wishes to study medicine" (p. 106).

James A. Sammons, Executive Vice President of the AMA, declares that "the AMA does not believe that there is an excess, nor would we agree to either the federal or state government intervening in the arbitrary determination of quotas of entry into the medical schools or into specialties of medicine" (p. 112). The AMA does support the upgrading of standards in residency programs, and recognizes that the growing competition in health care will affect doctors' incomes and their ability to set up practices. However, "the competition that bothers me is outside of medicine, among paramedicals that are springing up all over the place . . . in order to stabilize the system, we have to reduce the outside competitors for the inside quality of medicine" (p. 110).

With respect to FMGs, Dr. Sammons favors rigorous testing for all candidates for licensure, but "I would have a great deal of difficulty with the concept that U.S. citizens could be denied their right to return home and pursue their chosen field simply because they did not stay here" (p. 111).

(B) Articles

105. Ahmad, Busharat. "FMGs Have Good Reason to Participate in Organized Medicine." *Michigan Medicine* 85(10) (October 1986): 536.

Dr. Ahmad addresses the AMA's new emphasis on supporting foreign medical graduates (FMG) and soliciting their membership in the Association. The author references the AMA's Board of Trustees and their Ad Hoc Committee on FMGs. Ahmad says the Committee made 30 recommendations which call on FMGs to become active participants in organized medicine. The article points out that AMA policy opposes discrimination against race, creed, color, national origin or medical school. Furthermore, the Association opposes the use of accreditation standards to regulate physician manpower.

106. Akin, Rush. "Alabama Housestaff Looks at the AMA." *Journal of the Medical Association of the State of Alabama* 45(2) (August, 1975): 13-14.

Dr. Rush attended an annual AMA convention and, with a better understanding of the Association, calls on young doctors to support the AMA and their initiatives to support the interests of physicians. Rush claims that the typical medical school does not expose the student to the AMA nor the advantages of joining state and local medical societies. He maintains the Association offers low dues to interns and residents and that the House of Delegates has voting members who represent housestaff interests. Dr. Rush says the AMA is effectively doing its part to fight the malpractice insurance war, to push for legislation that precludes socialized medicine, and much much more. "It is now up to the young physicians," says Rush, "to appreciate what potential the AMA holds...and (be) the effective champion of our right to practice medicine as we have known it."

107. "AMA Aims to Pilot RCT Project in Four Sites." *American Journal of Nursing* (December 1988): 1717-1720.

This short article provides an excellent example of a battle between the AMA and other health care associations over a critical issue impacting the entire country. The nation's acute shortage of nurses led the AMA to propose that some be designated as "Registered Care Technologists (RCT)." This technologist would undergo 9-18 months of training and be certified to perform certain tasks now assigned to nurses. While the initiative eventually failed as a solution to the nursing shortage, the issue is exemplary of AMA's concern for adequate manpower in all health care professions.

108. Anlyan, William G. "What Has Happened to the AAMC Since the Coggeshall Report of 1965?" *Journal of American Medical Association* 210(10) (December 8, 1969): 1897-1900.

In 1964, the Executive Council of the Association of American Medical Colleges (AAMC) authorized "an ad hoc committee" under Dr. Lowell Coggeshall to "study and make recommendations regarding the future objectives, structure and function of the AAMC." Coggeshall issued his report in April, 1965, which, among other actions, recommended restructuring of the AAMC. By 1969, the resulting changes led to an organization more representative of the major components of medical schools. The revamped organization was also more effective in interfacing with other educational and research activities, the federal government, the AMA, practicing physicians, medical students, college students and others.

109. Barzun, Jacques. "The Professions Under Siege." *Harper's* (October, 1978): 61-66, 68.

The author, as Professor Emeritus at Columbia University, warns that medicine as a profession is approaching the same negative state of popular reputation as law. Barzun cautions doctors are increasingly seen as "only investing in money", covering up for one another's homicidal mistakes and engaging in lobbying which inhibits the advent of a much-improved national health system. The author maintains that any profession is a vulnerable institution which can be destroyed or destroy itself very rapidly. Barzun says a democracy, bent on equality in all things, will judge any profession by its worst exemplars. He charges the modern professions with having enjoyed their monopolies for so long that they have forgotten that it is a privilege given in exchange for a public benefit. "The message for the professions today is that their one hope of survival with anything like their present freedoms is the recovery of mental and moral forces." If doctors do not effectively police themselves without thought to public relations, it will be taken over by government. Yet policing is not enough. Doctors must "feel once more confident that ethical behavior is desirable, widely practiced, approved and admired." In short, a surviving profession today must ensure that competence and morality remain strong.

110. Burda, David. "Nurse Groups Oppose AMA: Plan to Create New Class of Workers." *Modern Healthcare* (July 1, 1988): 5.

This very short article by David Burda provides the American Nursing Association (ANA) perspective of the AMA proposal to create Registered Care Technologists (RCTs). The ANA claimed the AMA sought to gain more control over nursing by having RCTs report to physicians. In addition, the ANA said that the AMA hoped RCTs would alleviate the nursing shortage which has forced hospitals to close beds and has lessened physician income. Finally, the ANA said the RCT plan would duplicate roles, create low-skilled, low-paid positions that would be hard to fill, and jeopardize the quality of patient care. The RCT issue is an excellent example of how organized medicine can encounter significant resistance when it seeks to foster a major change in health care structure, policy, and process.

111. Burrows, Seymour J. "Negotiation - A New Dimension in AMA Activity." *Connecticut Medicine* 43 (6) (June 1979): 385-387.

This article describes the AMA's Department of Negotiations which was formed to increase member knowledge of negotiation techniques, establish state, local and medical specialty society negotiating structures and assist societies and physicians with specific problems requiring negotiation. The department sponsors seminars and institute training in the negotiation process and provides consultant services to individual physicians and groups of physicians.

112. Butter, Irene and Rebecca G. Sweet. "Licensure of Foreign Medical Graduates (FMG): A Historical Perspective." *Health and Society* 55 (Spring 1977): 315-340.

The authors trace the changes in U.S. federal and state legislation and licensure policy for FMGs since the 1920s. From 1953 to 1977, the number of FMGs in the U.S. increased sixfold and, in 1977, 20% of all practicing physicians in the U.S. were educated abroad. This dramatic increase resulted from liberalization of immigration policy to compensate for shortages in U.S. physicians, as well as the states gradually eliminating licensure restrictions that were unrelated to physician competency. Simultaneously, the states have adopted more standardized screening processes and more uniform qualification procedures. With the exception of the 1930s when the Great Depression struck the financial well being of most citizens, the AMA was supportive of FMGs attending U.S. medical schools. The Association furthermore compiled a list of approved foreign schools in the 1950s which many states then used for licensing decisions.

113. Canfield, Phillip R. "Family Medicine: A Historical Perspective." *The Journal of Medical Education* 51 (November 1976): 904-911.

Dr. Canfield's article traces the decline of general practitioners from the early 1900's and subsequently, the rise of Family Medicine through its approval as a new medical specialty in 1969. The author shows that fewer and fewer physicians were interested in comprehensive care, health maintenance, preventive medicine, rehabilitation, or the interaction between illness, environmental and psychological factors. Specializations multiplied as physician earnings increased substantially above general practitioners. Yet 85% of the ailments for which people consult physicians can be effectively handled by general practitioners.

Canfield shows how this trend reversed, with the concerted support of the AMA, American Academy of General Practice, Association of American Medical Colleges and World Health Organization. The role and training requirements of a newly defined "primary or personal physician" were established. These requirements called for another specialty with a distinct body of knowledge, requiring board certification. Unlike other specialty boards, these requirements specified certification for six years, thereafter requiring recertification. After 1969, the numbers of doctors entering Family Practice grew substantially, helping to offset losses incurred in the shortage of general practitioners.

114. Chapman, Carleton B. "On the Definition and Teaching of the Medical Ethics." *The New England Journal of Medicine* 301 (12) (September 20, 1979): 630-634.

This excellent article by Dr. Chapman reviews medical ethics from Hippocrates, London's College of Physicians, Thomas Percival and the AMA. Chapman claims, ethics to date have been little more than rules and etiquette to promote the good of the profession and its organization.

Nowhere do these statements focus on a patient-centered ethics and affirm the profession's commitment to it. Dr. Chapman claims a new ethics would better guide physicians, as well as help alleviate negative public opinion which perceives the medical profession as "acting unaimously in its own interest."

115. Crowley, Anne E. "Highlights of the 1989 Education Issue." *Journal of the American Medical Association* 262 (8) (August 25, 1989): 1001-1002.

The *JAMA* produces an excellent Education Issue each year which provides statistics, trends, and related data regarding medical schools in the U.S. Such issues, as this one cited, include facts on medical school enrollment, finance, graduate medical education, continuing medical education, foreign medical school graduates, and allied health education.

116. Domescik, Judy. "AMA - ERF - Ensuring Quality Medical Education." *Journal of MAG* 79 (April 1990): 227-228.

This article describes the purposes, fund raising mechanisms and benefits derived from the AMA's Education and Research Foundation (AMA - ERF). The Foundation, over 36 years old, was established to foster quality education in the nation's medical schools. AMA - ERF provides monies for four basic funds which go to medical schools as purely discretionary money or tagged for student financial aid, experimental health and medical programs and specific research areas. The AMA Auxiliary, comprised of spouses of AMA physician members, is a prime fund raiser for the Foundation. Of special effectiveness is the Auxiliary's state and local initiatives to raise tax free donations through auctions, raffles, parties, in memoriam donations and sharing cards. The AMA -ERF has proved most effective, distributing more than $49 million in loans since 1950, as well as over $1 million in gifts yearly.

117. Egan, Richard L. "The AMA, Accreditation, and the Number of Physicians." *Journal of American Medical Association* 230 (1974): 1681-1682.

This brief article is representative of the AMA's denial of charges that the Association limits the supply of doctors through manipulating standards and policies of medical schools. Dr. Egan claims that the AMA, through its Council on Medical Education and participation in the Liaison Committee on Medical Education, fosters the expansion of medical schools as long as competent physicians are graduated.

118. Grouse, Lawrence. "AMA's 'Medicine Today' TV Program." *Journal of American Medical Association* 253 (1985): 2558-2559.

This brief editorial describes the AMA's "Medicine Today" program, which premiered on television January 6, 1985. The program is a half-hour of scientific and medical news for physicians, as well as coverage of key medical, legal, economic, and political events affecting medical practice. The program's treatment of controversial issues includes the AMA position as well as alternative points of view.

119. Haight, Fulton. "Law and Medicine, When Will the Hostage-Taking Cease?" *Vital Speeches* LV(6) (January 1, 1989): 180-185.

The speaker, an experienced attorney working closely with the medical profession in California, challenges doctors everywhere to organize and get active in combating the malpractice war. Haight accounts the important measures taken in California since 1975 and compares the results to other states like Florida and New York where malpractice liability can be five times that in California. Specifically, Haight challenges physicians to better discipline their own profession with state quality assurance boards and by getting tort reform legislation passed which restricts amounts of lawsuit recoveries, shortening the statute of limitations. The author also advises physicians to "rediscover their patients," taking time to know them again and discussing problems or mistakes candidly and honestly. This is an excellent example of how locally organized medicine can make a real difference in rooting out incompetence and better controlling a legal process that drives physicians out of practice.

120. Harmon, Robert G. "Intern and Resident Organizations in the United States: 1934-1977." *Health and Society* 56 (1978): 500-530.

The author traces the history of intern and resident organizations in their efforts to bargain for higher wages, shorter hours, the right to moonlight and reforms in health care institutions. In the process, some organizations, with a liberal focus, supported national health insurance, the end to discriminatory admissions policies in the medical schools and strikes by unorganized health care workers; accordingly, these liberal organizations were branded as exhibiting communist tendencies by the AMA and other conservatives. During the social activism of the 1960s, intern and resident associations often exposed inadequate patient care and working conditions to the media and public. Other more conservative groups received the support of the AMA as the latter sought to bolster membership. By the end of 1974, the AMA endorsed collective bargaining, angering many hospital administrators and medical school deans. By 1975, numerous studies were conducted by "house-staff" organizations across the U.S. This disruption led to numerous court judgments which debated intern and resident rights. Harmon concludes with an assessment on the impact of house-staff organization actions. The author maintains they were a major force behind improving salary and fringe benefits, and shorter hours and better working conditions. Harmon, however, says more costly house-staff then became replaced to some degree by physician assistants and their exposure of underfunded public hospitals often led to closures or staff cutbacks, thereby decreasing their own job potential. Finally, the author says these organizations will undoubtedly survive and "doctors will persist in seeking a strong voice in decision making through negotiated contracts."

121. Koska, Mary T. "AMA Offers New Service to Simplify Credentialing." *Hospitals* (December 5, 1990): 52.

Koska's article provides an excellent example of one of the many services the AMA can provide which is derived from their data base on all the nation's physicians. This new service is known as the National Physician Credentials Verification Service (NPCVS). The service will help hospitals, physicians and others who are working credentialing of medical staffs. For $50, the AMA will provide a NPCVS report which includes a doctor's personal history, education and training, liability insurance status, licenses, special board certificates, medical society membership, employment history and hospital affiliations.

122. Margolis, Richard J. "Why 117 Medical Schools Can't Be Right." *Change Magazine* (October 9/10, 1977): 26-33.

The author, Literary Editor of Change Magazine, provides a highly critical article regarding the AMA's "gatekeeping" via limitations on admissions to medical schools. Margolis claims the "sacred doctor-patient relationship so lovingly promoted by the AMA is now just a pleasant memory vanished in the wake of specialization, technology and third-party reimbursement." The author insists we must send to medical school those "who care" and in the numbers that will permit doctors to be "dispatched to all the land, . . . to sell federally financed health care at prices the nation can afford." Margolis examines past medical school entry history, policy and charges the AMA with promoting "policies which breed elitism and create artificial health care shortages." The author additionally claims the Medicare and Medicaid's "absurdly generous reimbursement policy, amounting to a blank check for doctors, was . . . the price the AMA exacted for allowing Medicare and Medicaid to pass." Skyrocketing physicians' incomes then triggered a boom in medical school enrollment and more corruption in the system to delimit a physician "surplus" which Margolis claims amounts to "a competitive situation in which doctors' incomes decline." Margolis calls for reform and basically a free market wherein the supply of doctors is not artificially influenced.

123. McNutt, David, R. "GMENAC: Its Manpower Forecasting Framework." AJPH 71(10) (October, 1981): 116-1124.

In this article, McNutt discusses the development of a manpower forecasting framework and series of models by the GMENAC that may have "significant utility in future human resource planning at both national and local levels." The GMENAC was chartered by the Department of Health and Human Services to "analyze the distribution among specialties of physicians and residents and evaluate alternative approaches to ensuring an approximate balance." The committee was organized into five working groups called Technical Panels which determine the physician manpower requirements for the decade up to 1990.

Several references were made to articles published in JAMA and other AMA resources. These include W.D. Holden's and E.J. Levitt's article on the migration of physicians from one specialty to another (JAMA, 1978; 239: 205-209), I. Jacoby's model of the Graduate Medical Education's impact on specialty distribution (JAMA, 1981; 245: 1046-1051), and P.C. Roddy's epidemiological based manpower requirements model (JAMA, 1980; 243: 355-358).

124. Mick, Stephen S. "The Foreign Medical Graduate." *Scientific American* 232(2) (February 1975) 14-15, 17, 19, 21.

The author accounts the significant rise of foreign medical graduates (FMG) in the U.S. since 1950. Factors include U.S. immigration laws and shortage of practitioners in the U.S. (at least into the 1970s). The article provides good statistics on points of origin, numbers of graduates, hospital staffing, specialty selections and more.

Negative aspects are addressed, such as the fact that third world providers of these graduates cannot offer them attractive employment or practicing conditions, and therefore have a deficit themselves of physicians. The author then shows available data is inadequate to make valid judgments regarding competency of the FMGs compared to graduates of U.S. medical schools. Unfortunately the FMG is often treated as substandard in the U.S. and perceived to be less competent. Mick charges "lacking a coherent policy regarding the numerous issues in medicine, the medical profession in the U.S. has allowed medical graduates to fill in the most obvious cracks in the system." This may now worsen a rising surplus, prevent other nations from solving medical manpower, and leaving the FMGs to fend for themselves.

125. Osteen, Arthur. "Licensure and International Medical Graduates." *Journal of the American Medical Association* 266(7) (August 21, 1991): 956-958.

This article describes the complexity of the issue of licensing international medical graduates (IMGs), otherwise termed foreign medical graduate (FMGs). As stated by the author, there have been at least 12 bills introduced in Congress since 1988 directed at prohibiting discrimination against graduates of foreign medical schools. Additionally, a recent study by the AMA found that anti-discrimination legislation was a primary goal for IMG organizations. The complexity of the issue is further exacerbated by the wide variation in laws and practices among the 50 states. To assist in easing some of the confusion over credentials assessment, the AMA offers the National Physician Credentials Verification Service for both IMGs and USMGs. Lastly the author clarifies the official AMA stance of firm opposition to federal intervention in the licensing process, and to discrimination based on race, ethnicity, or place of education.

126. Paxton, Robert E., and Walker, Frank B. "What Has the AMA Done for Me Lately?" *Michigan Medicine* (October 1986): 543-545.

The authors answer a question often heard by physicians, " What has the AMA done for me lately?" First and foremost, the AMA represents the medical profession to Congress, the White House, federal agencies, the courts, state government and others. The AMA recommends policy, provides testimony, lobbies specific interests and provides feedback on physician opinions. Moreover, the Association's General Counsel takes legal action to defend AMA interests in court.

Second, the AMA represents physicians in the malpractice insurance crisis. The Association drafted federal legislation to obtain state action on tort reform. The AMA published detailed information on this liability crisis and its costs to society. The Association additionally provides a dedicated "hot line" to advise physicians on liability questions.

Third, the AMA continues to provide significant scientific information and support for maintenance of high educational standards for physicians. The Association studies and reports on new medical technologies and procedures and their effectiveness and suitability for clinical use. The AMA proposes scientific initiatives and funds many of them. The Association's JAMA and specialty journals are published monthly. The AMA library and on-line data bases support members with information regarding all areas of medicine. The Association produces a weekly newspaper on socioeconomic events affecting medicine. The AMA also publishes its Home Health Library, Patient Medication Instruction sheets, and many other pamphlets, books and posters.

Fourth, AMA members can obtain current demographic information that supports decisions on where to practice or perhaps what specialty to pursue in a given area. Individual programs also offer AMA-sponsored insurance and retirement plans.

The article maintains that AMA members receive "plenty" in return for their annual dues. Specifically, the authors summarize benefits derived from AMA political lobbying and related representation of the profession. Next, the Association's actions to alleviate the medical malpractice liability "crisis" are reviewed. Legal actions by the AMA's General Counsel are also cited. The authors then account for the AMA's provision of scientific medical information and support of high medical education standards. A summary is provided on AMA publications, library services and the Diagnostic and Therapeutic Technology Assessment project. Finally, the article addresses services like provision of physician demographic data, the AMA Placement Service and insurance and retirement plans.

127. Pekas, Michael W. "Membership: It is a Question of Dollars and Sense." *South Dakota Journal of Medicine* (October, 1989): 11.

Dr. Pekas, as President of the South Dakota State Medical Association, calls on doctors to weigh the value of AMA rather than the price of its dues. The author says a good cost benefit analysis would make it clear that the AMA simply needs member support. Pekas summarizes tangible benefits as scientific publications, the *AM News*, educational seminars and workshops, insurance programs, and more. Intangible benefits include: representation of physicians' rights and interests to local, state and national government; the opportunity to define and monitor their own standards for medical education and care; and having a forum in which to raise issues, reach a consensus and formulate policy regarding diverse medical matters.

128. Pusey, William A. "Medical Education and Medical Service." *Journal of the American Medical Association* 84(4) (January 24, 1925): 281-285.

Dr. Pusey's article addresses the extreme shortage of general practitioners in U.S. cities and physicians of any type in rural areas. The author provides statistics from around the country that show more and more doctors are becoming specialists and that fewer physicians are willing to remain in rural areas. Those remaining in rural areas average more than fifty years old and the exodus continues. As a result, many remote areas are entirely without medical services. Moreover, nurses are increasingly required to perform physician tasks, and midwives are again growing rapidly to fill the vacuum. Dr. Pusey attributes much of the causes to making medical education so costly in time and money.

129. Reinhardt, Uwe E. "A Framework for Deliberations on the Compensation of Physicians." *Medical Practice Management* (Fall, 1987): 85-95.

The issue of physician reimbursement as a wage which not only represents the services provided by compensation for the physician's skill and time is addressed by Dr. Reinhardt in this article. He begins by asking what is an appropriate wage for a physician and what is the best method of payment. The statistics provided by the AMA in their Annual Survey of Physicians assisted the development of a recommendation to develop an alternative fee-for-service system based on negotiated fees.

130. Sammons, James H. "Health Manpower in the Medical Marketplace." *Health Affairs* 1(4) (Fall, 1992): 20-29.

Dr. Sammons, as Executive Vice President of the AMA, provides this excellent statement of the association's role and policy regarding health care manpower. Dr. Sammons explains two basic approaches taken in the past for managing health care manpower --the forecasting and planning approach and the market-oriented approach. The author maintains that many dynamic factors quickly impact the adequacy of manpower, to include new technologies, innovative practice management approaches, insurance industry decisions, government regulations, and general population movement. Dr. Sammons states that a supply and demand market oriented approach is much more effective in responding to these factors and in providing us the appropriate manpower. The article cites examples of government intervention that upset the proper balance of manpower.

Dr. Sammons then summarizes AMA policy: "The association has no desire to limit the production of properly trained physicians; the number of approved medical schools (should) be determined entirely by the ability of schools to meet acceptable educational standards; the use of incentives, education, encouragement and exhortation are infinitely preferable to prescription of numbers, types and location of physicians by legislation or regulation; medical school standards should not be adjusted to reflect changing socio-economic conditions; and the AMA will help physicians adjust to changing circumstances through the collection, analysis and dissemination of relevant information."

131. Seipp, Conrad. "Organized Medicine and the Public Health Institute of Chicago." *The Bulletin of Historical Medicine* 62 (1988): 429-449.

Conrad's article provides an example of how organized medicine vehemently fought contracted, salaried medicine at national, state and local levels. The author uses the case of a non-profit VD treatment center in Chicago and its experience with the Chicago Medical Society and AMA.

132. Steele, Mark M. "AMA Teaches Physicians to Fight Back." *Modern Healthcare* 6(1) (July, 1976): 31-34.

This article describes an AMA five-day seminar in negotiating. With physicians facing an ever rising batch of government legislation, hospital administrative challenges to the medical staff, or a battle with the insurance industry, doctors should learn negotiating skills. The AMA course includes value systems, the use of mediation, fact finding and related negotiating tools and techniques. In addition to the national association's courses, several state medical societies have formed their own departments of negotiators to prepare themselves for actions.

133. Stolfi, Julius E. "Thoughts on Continuing Medical Education." *New York State Journal of Medicine* 78(14) (December, 1978): 2247-2249.

This article accounts the rapid growth of continuing medical education (CME) in the United States and makes recommendations for improvement. By 1970, the AMA had designed and field-tested an accreditation program for CME which began 10 years earlier. The AMA's Council on Medical Education initiated accreditation at medical schools, specialty societies, government facilities, voluntary health organizations, state medical associations and community hospitals. In 1975, the Liaison Committee on Continuing Medical Education (LCCME) was founded by the AMA, the Association of American Medical Colleges, Council of Medical Specialty Societies, American Hospital Association and American Board of Medical Specialties. In July 1977, the LCCME became the only accrediting body in the U.S. for CME. The author shows that in the interim, many state medical societies, state boards of medical examiners, national medical specialty boards and societies made CME mandatory for membership, certification and re-certification. In 1975-76 alone, 119 medical schools provided 5,426 CME courses to over 300,000 physicians. The author calls on the LCCME to continue its management, streamlining and standardizing the accreditation process, cutting waste and duplication, and approving only those programs "which contribute factual, procedural and/or technical information to the practicing physician which can be used for the care of the sick."

134. Weithaus, Barbara and John J. Fauser. "Committee on Allied Health Education and Accreditation: Assessing Educational Outcomes and Assuring Quality." *Journal of the American Medical Association* 266(7) (August 21, 1991): 968-969.

This article reviews the role of the AMA Committee on Allied Health Education and Accreditation (CAHEA) in accreditation, assessment of educational outcomes, quality assurance, and the recognition of new occupations. Additionally, the scope of CAHEA influence in these areas is described. For example, the authors indicate that more than 33,000 entry-level professionals in 26 allied health disciplines graduate from CAHEA-accredited programs each year. The AMA sees the education of allied health professionals to work effectively with physicians as a primary mission of the CAHEA affiliated institutions and associations.

PRODUCTS AND SERVICES OF THE AMERICAN MEDICAL ASSOCIATION (AMA)

The AMA is a prolific producer of written literature, conferences, seminars, TV shows and radio broadcasts designed to support the physician and public consumers. The following items are representative of this output. For the latest guides to products and services, contact the Order Department, AMA, P. O. Box 2964, Milwaukee, WI 53201-2964, or phone 1 (800) 621-8335.

1. **Medical Education and Career Development**:

•*Medicine as a Career* (book). For college teachers and counselors to help students.
•*Medicine: A Chance to Make a Difference* (pamphlet). To help college students understand medical school admission requirements, how to choose a school, and other medical career factors.
•*Got that Healing Feeling* (pamphlet). To help high school students consider medical school entry.
•*Science and Art in the Name of Healing* (videotape). To help high school and college students consider Medicine as a career.
•*Twenty Eight Allied Health Careers* (book). Guide on physicians support professions and sources of further information.

•*Directory of Graduate Medical Education Programs* (book). Details in over 6,700 programs by Specialty.
AMA. Fellowship and Residency Electronic Interactive Database Access System (IBM software). An automatic aid to help find the best graduate training programs.
•*Allied Health Education Directory* (book). Guide to careers and over 2,500 education programs sponsored by more than 1,500 post-secondary institutions.

2. **Medical Practice:**

A. General Information

•*Fresh advice* (audio cassettes and booklet). Current practice planning and legal advice for physicians (two major topics).

•*American Medical News* (weekly tabloid newspaper). Provides scientific, social, political, and economic matters of significant importance to the medical community.

•*American Medical Television* (TV broadcast). A two-hour TV program on Sunday mornings. Discovery Channel, serving as a physician's continuing medical education program.

•*From Residency to Reality* (book). A practical manual for choosing a residency and marketing oneself for practice.

•*Physician Starter Pack I* (literature and videocassettes). An overall guide for starting your own practice. Pack II includes group practice.

•The AMA Medical Library (a service to physicians).
Supporting automated databases serves association members with with information on science, clinical medicine, health care administration and much more.

B. Legal

•*Physician's Survival Guide: Legal Pitfalls and Solutions* (book). Provides a reference guide by attorneys of the National Health Lawyers Association and AMA for physicians concerned with any legal matter.

•*AMA Medicolegal Forms with Legal Analysis.* (book). To assist physicians with patient relationships by providing guidance on recognizing legal liability and working with legal forms to cover these issues.

•*Annotated Current Opinions* (book). Covers court decisions and legal, medical, and health law articles which cite principles of medical ethics or current opinions on judicial affairs.

•*A Compendium of State Peer Review Immunity Laws* (book). Summarizes current laws affecting the peer review process.

•*AMA Tort Reform Compendium* (book). Provides state-by-state legislation and court rulings on tort reform and liability.

•*Grand Rounds on Medical Malpractice.* (book). A primary reference on the medical liability and risk management.

C. Ethics

•*The Constitution and Bylaws of the AMA* (booklet). Includes the current statement of AMA medical ethics, providing standards of conduct for doctors in their relationship with one another and with their patients.

•*Current Opinions* (booklet). Provides guidance for physicians on contemporary medical ethics by AMA's Council on Ethical and Judicial Affairs.

D. Reimbursement

•*Current Procedural Terminology (CPT)* (books, software, workshops, etc.). Various products to help report physician procedures and services to government and private insurance programs to expedite reimbursement.

•*International Classification of Diseases (ICD)* (books, software, and seminars). To help physicians with diagnosis codes needed for Medicare forms and billing statements.

•*Health Insurance Claim Forms* (forms and guidance booklets). To assist in making insurance claims.

•*Medical Collection Study Course* (audiocassette and workbook; also seminar). Guidance on how to expedite collection of overdue bills and increase office cash flow.

E. Communicating

•*AMA Manual of Style* (book). For physician authors; includes descriptions of on-line database resources.

•*Handling Patient Telephone Calls Effectively* (book and audiocassette). Physician's guide.

•*Patient Relations Guide* (booklet). Physician's guide.

•*Patient Survey Questionnaire* (forms). A preprinted questionnaire to obtain feedback from patients.

F. Physician Facts

•*American Medical Directory* (books or CD ROM disk). Provides demographics, credentials and professional data on all 600,000 plus physicians in the U.S. Data includes schooling, licensure information, specialty certification and any disciplinary actions. Data is derived from the AMA's Physician Masterfile maintained since 1906.

•*Physician Characteristics and Distribution in the U.S.* (booklet). Statistics and trends on physician distribution across the U.S.

•*Physician's Marketplace Statistics* (book). Primary reference on physician socioeconomic practice characteristics by geographical area.

•*AMA National (book).* Physician supply and utilization by specialty; trends and projections. Analysis of trends in physician manpower supply by specialty through 2010.

G. Special Populations.

•*HIV/AIDS Pack* (booklet and videocassette). To help the physician communicate with AIDS patients.

•*The Alcoholic Patient* (software). Physician's guide.

•*The Unresponsive Patient* (software). Physician's guide.

•*Adolescent Healthcare* (booklet). Use, costs, and problems of access. Statistics on prevention and treatment.

H. Business

•*The Business Side of Medical Practice* (booklet). Practice advice on all aspects of practice management.

•*Starting Your Practice Kit* (several booklets and checklists). Covers valuing practices, financing, timetables and business guidance.

•*The Complete Medical Marketing Handbook* (booklet and worksheets). A physician's guide.

•*Enhancing the Value of Your Medical Practice* (booklet). How-to guide on startup, expansion, mergers, acquistions, financing, joint ventures, and retirement plans.

•*Group Practice Kit* (several booklets). Guidance on forming or joining a partnership or group practice.

•*Planning Guide for Physician's Medical Facilities* (booklet). Guidance on location, design, construction, purchase, rental, and more.

•*Closing Your Practice* (booklet). Guidance on practical, legal and medical considerations.

•*Gearing Up for Retirement* (Seminar workbook). Practical guidance with forms and checklists.

3. **Scientific Medical Information:**

•*The Journal of the American Medical Association* (JAMA) (weekly magazine). This is the very "heart" of the AMA, providing the world's most widely read medical journal. The scientific and medical information of JAMA is published in seven foreign languages and distributed in 132 countries. JAMA provides basic science, research and treatment trends, as well as clinical and investigative reports on the latest specialty developments.

•*Drug Evaluation Annual* (annual, book or magazine subscription). Comprehensive physician's guide on the use of prescription drugs.

Nine Specialty Journals

American Journal of Diseases of Children
Archives of Dermatology
Archives of General Psychology
Archives of Internal Medicine
Archives of Neurology
Archives of Ophthalmology
Archives of Otolaryngology
Archives of Pathology and Laboratory Medicine
Archives of Surgery

4. **Consumer Medical Information:**

•*AMA Family Medicine Guide* (book). AMA's best selling volume on general ailments which family members can hopefully recognize, understand and obtain treatment.
•*AMA Handbook of First Aid and Emergency Care* (book). An excellent illustrated primer on emergency care "how to".
•*How to Understand Your Symptoms* (book). Superb, fully illustrated text to help you diagnose your illness and more smartly seek medical care. Separate editions exist for children, men and women.
•*AMA Handbook of Poisonous and Injurious Plants* (book). Promotes rapid diagnosis and treatment for poisons from plants or chemicals.
•*Sex Talk for a Safe Child* (booklet). A coloring book to teach young children about their bodies and preventing abuse.
•In addition to these and many other books, the AMA sponsors the American Medical Radio News, providing daily interviews with scientists and doctors. This program is available to all radio stations in the U.S. AMA additionally provides the nation's editors with weekly information packets based on AMA journal articles. Furthermore, the AMA's public information department fields daily queries from the media, answering questions on all aspects of health and AMA activities.

5. **Legislative matters:**

•*Textbook of Legislation* (book). Provides medical students an introduction to the legislative process, congressional internships for medical students, and how physicians can get actively involved.
•*Congressional Directory* (booklet). Provides names, addresses, and phone numbers of Congressional Contacts for healthcare matters.

•*Your Day on Capitol Hill - AMA National Education Conference* (conference). Introduces physicians to the legislative process and how doctors can become active in the process.

6. **Policy:**

•*AMA Policy Compendium* (book). Provides a thorough description of approximately 2,000 AMA policies which are readily referenced by topic.
•*Compendium of Political Strategies* (booklet). Addresses issues and trends using practical lessons on politics for developing political skills.
•*Use of Animals in Biomedical Research* (pamphlet). Covers the philosophical and moral issues as well as the need for and benefits of using animals in medical research.

7

POLICY AND POLITICAL ACTIVITIES AND ISSUES

The political and policy activities and perspectives of the American Medical Association are the primary topic of the readings contained in this chapter. The great influence of the AMA (described in an earlier chapter) largely came from the organization's political skill. As several of the readings covered below point out, the AMA was by no means free of internal tensions and conflicts of all sorts. Nevertheless, the Association (more so than almost any other interest group in U.S. history) was able to advance its own policy vision and see it enacted into national public policy.

As an organization representing upper middle class and largely politically conservative physicians, the AMA above all has fought to preserve physician domination of health care management, and physician autonomy with respect to treatment. It has resisted the rising influence of payor groups within health care, feeling (with justification) that this influence would sooner or later reduce the effective power and independence of doctors. Nevertheless, when health care reforms did come about (as with Medicare and Medicaid), the Association was effective in steering policy implementation in a favorable manner. The AMA has even indicated its willingness to support some forms of national health insurance - as long as the resulting program did not disturb the dominant position of physicians within the health care system itself.

Critics of the AMA see many negative results flowing from the system that the AMA has supervised. Care has been more forthcoming for the well-to-do, while the poor have been neglected. Unlike medical service systems in Western Europe (for example), the U.S. system reinforces a dominant capitalist class, and indeed becomes a chief ally of the rich and powerful. The AMA has also jealously guarded its privileges by unfairly attacking nonphysician providers (osteopaths and chiropractors, for example) as "quacks" and "cults". Other analysts, however, credit the AMA with some worthy achievements in policy areas such as medical education and public health.

A number of the books and articles deal more directly with the internal politics of the Association. As they show, there is no longer a general consensus among physicians as to what functions the AMA should fulfill, and the policies it should support. The organization has some physician critics who say it has become too passive and accepting of governmental activism, while others complain that AMA is too inflexible and reactionary.

There are disagreements within the national organization, and between the national organization and various state chapters. All in all, the readings here demonstrate that even the most powerful and successful interest groups in the U.S. will begin to experience internal conflicts during periods of uncertainty and stress. Like the rest of the nation, the AMA has been affected by the winds of change buffeting the health care system.

(A) Books

135. American Medical Association. *1846 - 1958 Digest of Official Actions.* Chicago, IL: American Medical Association, 1959.

This book is a complete collection of official (passed by the House of Delegates) American Medical Association policy positions. In the Introduction, Susan Crawford states that "the purpose of this volume is to provide a basic reference tool which will serve as a guide to both current and past policies" (p. 3). The book has 751 pages of text, an appendix (listing each AMA president, term of office, secretary, treasurer, date of annual meeting, and place of meeting), and an extensive index.

The work is organized like an encyclopedia, with topics arranged alphabetically. Within many topics, there are further subdivisions, and AMA House of Delegates policies regarding each topic are covered in chronological order. Descriptions of policy resolutions range from one paragraph to a page in length. In addition, a specific citation (date and page reference within the Official Proceedings of the House of Delegates) for each activity is provided after the description. Official policies published in the Journal of the American Medical Association are also covered.

136. Birenbaum, Arnold. *Health Care and Society.* Montclair, NJ: Allanheld, Osmun and Co., 1981.

According to the author, "in this book, health care is examined from the point of view of a sociologist looking at institutional development, the forces for change, and the unanswered challenges that remain" (p.x). Fifteen chapters and 250 pages of text are divided into four parts. In Part One, Birenbaum's sociological approach is described. "The Social Structure of Health Services", including the profession of medicine, is outlined in Part Two. In "Changing Patterns of Health Services" (Part Three), new educational practices, professional identities and practitioner conflicts are explored. The author concludes his work by studying "Emerging Social Issues", including the women's health movement and the concept of "health care with a human face".

Birenbaum analyzes American Medical Association activities, and concludes that the group is quite powerful, primarily through its successful efforts to maintain doctors' professional autonomy. "One of the AMA's tasks is to guard the rights of physicians. Efforts by other health care practitioners to increase their responsibilities are often met with hostility by the AMA, except where the tasks are specifically turned over to others by physicians" (p. 83). He cites the long- standing conflict between the AMA and chiropractors as an example. In the author's opinion, the AMA is much less willing to support any effective supervision of physician practices that might be considered unethical.

There are signs, however, that the extensive autonomy of physicians, particularly since the inaction of Medicare and Medicaid, may in fact lead to supervisory policies that the AMA most opposes. "It is ironic that the original resistance to state regulation of Medicare and Medicaid by the AMA has permitted the growth of routine deviation in the field and has set the groundwork for even more control than was originally anticipated" (p. 93). The new institutional payers in health care (including the Federal Government) are increasingly willing to alter the traditional notions of physician autonomy in their efforts to control costs.

As a consequence, doctors are steadily losing power within the health care system. Despite AMA opposition, physicians have diminishing power to set fees, and chiropractors are eligible for Medicare and Medicaid reimbursement. In the not-so-distant future, "broad-based support for further social change could emerge after a vigorous conflict between the advocates of a national health service and the opposition, led by the AMA, the American Hospital Association, and drug manufacturers" (p.236). The establishment of "health care with a human face" will mean greater emphasis on patient, not physician, autonomy and responsibility.

137. Cater, Douglas and Philip R. Lee. *Politics of Health.* New York, NY: Medcom Press, 1972.

Cater and Lee, as editors, have compiled a book composed of a series of lectures and seminars on the politics of health. Mr. Cater, as former Special Assistant to President Johnson for health programs, stated that "politics is too important to be left to the generals" (p. 1). Reflecting on how political forces of the nation shape the future of health care in America, he expresses the need to create health policy centers for developing plans and measuring performance and broadening the horizons of health professionals which will facilitate the development of a national health strategy.

The authors of this collection mention the AMA's role in the development of health policies. As health lobbyist, Paul D. Ward states that "the AMA has acquired the primary public image of being a crusader against national health insurance" (p. 38). The specifics of the AMA's political influences is presented in the piece by Dwight L. Wilbur, M.D., "The AMA in Washington." As past president of the AMA, Dr. Wilbur discusses the achievements and failures of the AMA as a lobbying group over such issues as national health insurance and the Medicare legislation.

138. Califano, J. A. Jr. *America's Health Care Revolution.* New York, NY: Random House, 1986.

This is a policy-oriented, lay-person's examination of the changes in the U.S. health care system in the last twenty-five years. The author is a veteran policymaker who addressed health care cost, quality and access concerns under Presidents Lyndon Johnson (as Special Assistant for Domestic Affairs) and Jimmy Carter (Secretary of Health, Education and Welfare, now Health and Human Services), and Lee Iacocca at Chrysler Motor Corporation. Now working as an influential lawyer in Washington, D.C., Califano has reflected upon his experiences in this brief (eleven chapters and 225 pages) and simply-written book.

In Califano's opinion, the American Medical Association has done well for its members by doing good. Through the efforts of the AMA (along with other groups), medical education was upgraded and pure food and drug legislation was enacted. On the other hand, the power that physicians gained over the marketplace through such laws was used to restrict competition and enrich doctors. To get to this position of control, the AMA focused on political organization. "Organized along state lines, the association created potent political action groups, alerted the public to the false claims of many patent medicines, and became a force to reckon with in the legislative and regulatory process, national and local" (p. 38).

After initial misgiving, the AMA came around to support the use of private health insurance--the beginning of a "money tree" that doctors took full advantage of. National health insurance was a much different matter. "The AMA was ready to fight in 1945, when President Truman proposed a sweeping national health insurance program. . . . In 1949 and 1950 the AMA spent $2.8 million in a massive public relations campaign that effectively branded Truman's national health insurance proposal as socialized medicine" (p. 49). By the 1984 Congressional elections, the AMA's political action committee was contributing $3 million to friendly candidates.

The AMA has meticulously protected the financial well-being of its members, often opposing reform proposals such as second- opinion programs for surgery and HMO subsidization. From his vantage point as a Johnson Administration insider, Califano describes the opposition to Medicare by the AMA and others. The program was finally enacted, but with costly compromises that permitted the payment of "customary" and "prevailing" physicians' fees. "Johnson accepted this system to blunt AMA claims that government would control doctors' fees. . . . As a result, physicians would gain even greater power to charge what the traffic would bear" (p. 52).

The author believes that the rapid evolution of our health care system since the introduction of Medicare and Medicaid in 1965 can be fairly termed a "revolution". Given such factors as the demographic "graying of America" and accelerating technological innovation, the U.S. is facing unprecedented financial, legal and ethical problems. There is a high level of waste within some areas of our health care system, while other places are starved for resources. At the same time, though, Califano sees the potential for meeting these challenges with the right combination of public policy, corporate innovation, and public education.

139. Campion, Frank, D. *The AMA and U.S. Health Policy Since 1940*. Chicago, IL: Chicago Review Press, 1984.

This book is a comprehensive review and analysis of the participation of the American Medical Association in national health care policy making since 1940. It is an authorized history (approved by the AMA Board of Trustees, and written by a former AMA employee), but Frank Campion attempts to provide a balanced view of the political controversies engaging the AMA in modern times. Research sources include the proceedings of the AMA House of Delegates, interviews with AMA notables, and a wide range of other historical and political documents.

The book is organized into four parts (Environment, Organization, Events and Interfaces). The first part is an overview of the major scientific and technological breakthroughs that revolutionized health care in the first part of the Twentieth Century, including advances in pharmacology and surgical procedure. As the title indicates, Part Two describes the basic organizational structures and processes of the AMA, in particular the functioning of the House of Delegates. It analyzes how the operations of the AMA have been affected by the ongoing evolution in physician training and professional identity. Campion also explains how the AMA attempts to reflect physician needs and concerns through its varied scientific, educational and professional representation activities.

Campion's account of the AMA's involvement in public policy controversies really begins in Part Three (Events). Campion suggests that, until the 1940s, the American Medical Association and its members were almost completely absorbed in the scientific and technological revolution in health care, and how it was changing physician capabilities and duties. The AMA's efforts to reorganize and upgrade U.S. medical education along scientific lines (which included but by no means was limited to implementing the recommendations of the Flexner Report) had been highly successful. The political revolution that began with Franklin Roosevelt's New Deal in the 1930s, however, brought into question the dominant national vision of a physician-supervised and private sector-oriented health care system.

In Campion's view, neither the AMA nor its physician members were-well prepared for this challenge. Indeed, it is repeatedly suggested throughout this section of the book that physicians are deeply ambivalent about the organization-building and politically-oriented activities essential for success in the policy arena. Physicians are portrayed as idealists searching for ever-increasing clinical certainty and precision in their professional activities--behavior patterns that do not often transfer well to the political arena. Consequently, physicians have often responded to political criticism with an intense self-righteousness that worked against their own interests in a policy making process requiring compromise and coalition-building.

Nevertheless, with the help of a series of ideological and economic allies and advisors (including conservative, pro-business Republicans and shrewd public relations managers such as Clem Whitaker and Leone Baxter), the AMA was able to sidetrack the most sweeping proposals for health care reform in the 1940s and 1950s, such as the Wagner-Murray-Dingell plan for national health insurance. The Sixties, however, showed the limitations of the customary AMA approach. Its image as a rigid and shrill opponent of national health programs led to an erosion of public support, while more articulate spokespersons for governmental involvement in health care (such as Presidents Kennedy and Johnson) were skillfully presenting their case to the public. As a result, the AMA coalition was decisively defeated in Washington with the passage of legislation establishing the Medicare and Medicaid programs in 1965.

Campion suggests that this defeat was in fact a blessing in disguise for the AMA. It prompted the rise of new and more pragmatic leadership. By focusing more on political action, and the details of regulation and policy implementation in Washington, the AMA was able to play an influential role in the actual design of Medicare and Medicaid. Operating with much greater political sophistication, and aided by rapidly increasing public skepticism about the cost and effectiveness of large Federal Government programs, the organization once again successfully worked to derail a drive for national health insurance (spearheaded by Senator Edward Kennedy, a younger brother of the late President).

With a slowdown in economic growth, and escalating yearly increases in health care costs, American health care entered an era of limits. The "politics of rising costs" (as Campion terms it) cut both ways. On the one hand, it worked to discourage additional efforts by government to provide health care services. On the other hand, efforts at cost containment inevitably began focusing on the roles and rewards the physician possessed within the health care system. Compounding the AMA's difficulties was an organizational crisis in finance that lasted through much of the 1970s. It took vigorous membership drives, substantial dues increases, budgetary cutbacks, and structural modifications, to restore financial solvency. (To take one example, the number of councils and committees in the AMA was reduced from 68 to 8 at the 1975 annual meeting.) Once again, however, Campion concludes that the AMA in fact strengthened itself, since its responses transformed the organization into a more centralized and streamlined operation that could better meet the new challenges of the 1980s.

The final section of the book, Interfaces, focuses on the AMA's historical and current activities in education and science, including often-controversial policy issues such as FMGs and the growing clinical responsibilities of the allied health professions. It also provides a concise account of the development of AMA specialty journals, and the efforts made to keep the *Journal of the American Medical Association* a premier medical publication.

Campion's summary view of the impact of the association on modern American health care is largely positive. While agreeing with AMA and physician critics that motives of economic self-interest have not been absent in the various efforts to reform medicine and physician training, Campion nevertheless suggests that "physicians are more strongly motivated by their pride in being a doctor and their sense of professional responsibility" (p. 432), and the AMA "has clearly worked in the medical interests of the American people" (p. 514). As cost containment efforts continue to dominate the functioning of the health care system in the 1980's and beyond, and systemic reorganization proposals continue to gain national attention, Campion is confident that the AMA can continue to evolve in response, working to preserve a high-quality and primarily non-governmental administered system.

140. DeGroot, Leslie J., Editor. *Medical Care: Social and Organizational Aspects*. Springfield, IL: Thomas, 1966.

This book was compiled from articles by various writers published in the New England Journal of Medicine from July, 1963 through February, 1964 dealing with the medical profession's problem of organizing and distributing medical service.

In chapter thirty, "The American Medical Association," by Norman A. Welch, M.D. (deceased) and D.F. Ward, M.D., the authors look at the AMA's twin goals "To promote the science and art of medicine and the betterment of public health" as well as how the AMA has pursued these goals since its birth in 1847. The authors describe the AMA's national policy-making body, the House of Delegates (over 225 members including delegates elected from constituent associations), each of the twenty sections of the AMA's Scientific Assembly, each of the government services and the student AMA.

Welsh and Ward go on to review AMA programs and activities that affect the practice of medicine. One of the greatest activities is its publications such as the *Journal of the American Medical Association* (JAMA), published since 1883, specialty journals, reference books, medical newspapers, and various pamphlets and reports. Its publications make it one of the leaders in scientific publishers. The AMA also sponsors scientific meetings during which members gather and evaluate data on new products, new findings and new methods. There are councils on drugs, food, nutrition, and medical education. It maintains these committees based on current interests and demands. It inaugurated and administers a medical student loan program and represents the profession in Washington.

The authors believe that the AMA serves the public and for over a century has delivered itself to the unselfish ideals embodied in its constitution by the Founding Fathers. The physician members of this organization have reason to be proud of the AMA, its dedication, its work, and its accomplishments.

141. Ehrenreich, Barbara, and John Ehrenreich. *The American Health Empire.* New York, NY: Random House, 1970.

"If this book can be said to have a single thesis, it is that the American health system is not in business for people's health" (p. vii). The authors, noted and outspoken political liberals, are members of the Health Policy Advisory Center (Health-PAC), a New York City-based advocacy group. They see the U.S. health care system as dominated by professional elites that primarily work for the best interests of American capitalism and the economic upper classes. They call for "radical social change" - the democratic restructuring of health care. The titles of the nineteen chapters of the book ("The Blue Cross We Bear," "Medicaid: Killers of the Dream," and "The Empire Has No Clothes") clearly express their viewpoint.

The American Medical Association is portrayed as the chief power center for elitist and plutocratic health policy in the "medical-industrial complex," and a major obstacle to rationalizing the health care system. The AMA prevents medical school expansion, thus contributing to the shortage of doctors. However, the authors also suggest that the Association's power was at its highest in the Forties and Fifties. Now the AMA has lost political influence to other elements of the medical elite-- hospitals, equipment and pharmaceutical companies, and insurers, in particular. The era of the physician, and the AMA, is coming to an end. "The battles go on, but the war is over. . . . While the AMA pours its money into symbolic battles and public relations face-lifting, the empires are steadily, confidently building. There is no going back for the American health care system . . . . The age of the guild-dominated, individual medical craftsman is over" (p. 39).

The authors elsewhere refer to the AMA's political efforts as "pathetic" and "rear-guard" (p. 48). The initiatives produced by the Association tend to be defensive in nature, and are offered to coopt more effective and systemic reforms. (The AMA proposals for national health insurance fall into this category.)

142. Fox, Daniel M. *Health Policies, Health Politics.* Princeton, NJ: Princeton University Press, 1986.

Dr. Fox, a Professor at the State University of New York, Stony Brook, provides the reader with a comparative account of health politics and policymaking in the United States and Britain between 1911 and 1965. Unlike many (perhaps most) authors, Dr. Fox focuses on the similarities rather than differences in national policies. It is his view (put forth in eleven chapters spanning two hundred pages) that both the U.S. and U.K. are now facing unexpected (and often unpleasant) results of the policy he terms "hierarchical regionalism"--in essence, an overreliance upon established medical research and delivery systems.

In the author's view, the American Medical Association's policy positions and political activities reflected internal contradictions and professional ambivalence as often as a self-assured unanimity. The perceived threat of the Committee on the Costs of Medical Care (CCMC) report temporarily unified most AMA physicians in opposition to "socialized medicine." By the fifties, however, there was a growing split in attitudes and interest between generalists and specialists within the AMA. The dominant generalists in solo practice combined with other AMA members who were uncomfortable with his personal style to oust Morris Fishbein, the powerful leader of the Association. The generalists tended toward a nostalgia for the "old-fashioned" doctor who worked alone, and felt threatened by the rise of specialized, hospital-based practice.

The Association did succeed in supporting many winning political candidates (usually Republicans such as Everett Dirksen in 1950 and Dwight Eisenhower in 1952). However, "the AMA's political effectiveness was as much a result of the problems of the New Deal coalition as of the power of organized medicine" (p. 156). The postwar swing to conservatism facilitated the defeat of Fair Deal proposals for health care insurance and regulations that the AMA termed "socialized medicine." But "the AMA's tactics . . . were successful when opposing interest groups mobilized their strength" (p. 158).

Despite AMA indifference or hostility, Federal government involvement in biomedical research and medical education increased steadily during the fifties. Despite the AMA's strongly held belief in physician independence, it felt compelled to accept the growing influence of academic and hospital-based doctors. Indeed, seeing the possibility of governmental subsidies, the Association reversed its previous position and agreed that there was a grave danger of a physician shortage. The resulting educational expansion increased the number of physicians, but also fueled continuing Federal involvement in health care.

By the sixties, old-style AMA opposition to governmental involvement in health care had in effect disappeared. The Association's attempt to stop the inaction of Medicare and Medicaid was doomed, since the growing nationalization of medical care ensured that only some details, not the general principles, of the programs were still in question. With the inauguration of Medicare and Medicaid, "hierarchical regionalism" had triumphed.

143. Friedson, Eliot. *Professional Dominance: The Social Structure of Medical Care*. New York, NY: Atherton Press, Inc., 1970.

"Health services are organized around professional authority, and their basic structure is constituted by the dominance of a single profession over a variety of other, subordinate occupations" (p. xi). This assertion, taken from the Foreword, best summarizes both Eliot Friedson's focus of study and key operating assumption. Friedson, a medical sociologist at New York University, explores the role of professionalism in health services provision, and suggests how reorganized medical care might provide greater responsiveness to patient needs. With a great emphasis on linking the concept of health care professionalism to the larger realm of sociological theory (the ideas of Karl Marx, Max Weber and Talcott Parsons, among others, appear repeatedly), this complex work is more useful to a basic social theorist or researcher than someone concerned with gathering empirical information on the actual impact of professions on health services delivery.

This reasonably concise book (somewhat over two hundred pages) is organized into an Introduction ("Substantive Issues in Medical Sociology") and three parts, covering nine chapters. In "A Sociological Approach to Medical Care", Friedson criticizes what he sees as the underdeveloped and medical profession-oriented field of medical sociology, and calls for more independent analysis. He offers "A Structural Approach to Medical Care", which focuses on the environment rather than the individual as the object of analysis, and hypothesizes that the social structure of profession largely determines the nature of medical practice.

In Part 2, Friedson examines "The Position of the Profession in the Medical Care Structure" in greater detail. Concentrating on the physician, he emphasizes the factor of professional dominance in the design of medical education and practice as the critical factor in controlling clinical performance. Despite the range of practice modes (from solo fee-for-service to more bureaucratized group practices), Friedson sees clinical performance and, more importantly, mindset as largely standardized. The medical profession can permit a great deal of functional autonomy, but only if techniques and judgment are professionally established beforehand.

The effect of all of this is to turn the physician profession into a "priesthood." Patients, like parishioners, are admonished to have faith, and to obey. Other health care professions are arranged in a descending hierarchy of subordination. Most importantly, the patient is left in ignorance, and depersonalized and distanced from his or her own treatment. For this problem, Friedson prescribes less professional autonomy, and greater control by the surrounding medical bureaucracies (the hospital, the university, and so forth) and their administrators.

Friedson does not directly respond to the inevitable "from the frying pan into the fire" objections to his proposal that come to mind. Instead, he begins Part 3 by arguing that control of professionals through "rationalization" of services has already taken place in manufacturing, and many other service industries, and probably will do so in health care as well. This rationalization need not be too bad for the patient if it is combined with an emphasis on greater patient participation in the particulars of her or his own care, and greater concern for the humanistic side of health services. Nevertheless, some depersonalization is inevitable given the nature of a hospital. Therefore, Friedson concludes, the most important thing may be to minimize the use of hospital services, and shift more care into ambulatory settings. He sees these as being amenable to greater patient and less professional control.

In his concluding chapter ("Professional Dominance and the Reorganization of Medical Care"), Friedson calls for a process of medical care that is "a personal service to human beings who have the right to the dignified status of adults who participate in determining what happens to them" (p. 210). Along these lines, he offers five reorganization principles for health care: 1) reduce health care professional autonomy and self-regulation; 2) build up a bureaucratic system to provide a "check" on professional activity; 3) take care, however, that such bureaucratic mechanisms are themselves limited and "checked"; 4) increase the patient's "voice in the organization, presentation, and substance of the care he gets" (p. 215); and 5) patient participation mechanisms should emphasize individuals rather than groups. Given that Friedson's work is now dated and quite general when it comes to actual policy measures, however, the reader will have to rely more upon other sources of information to follow through on the theoretical vision provided within.

144. Garceau, Oliver. *The Political Life of the American Medical Association.* Cambridge, MA: Harvard University Press, 1961.

Though now obviously dated, this book was a landmark study of the internal politics of the American Medical Association when it appeared. Its author, a Professor in Harvard University's Department of Government, divides his short (175 text pages) analysis into five chapters: "Political Morphology: The Forms of Political Life"; "Political Histology: the 'Active Minority'"; Political Physiology: The Process of Governing in the Association"; "Political Pathology:

Tension in the Association"; and "Political Ecology: Group and Community". Dr. Garceau explores AMA organizational behavior through application of "group theory", a major analytical framework within political science that was later subsumed into more and more general political theory of pluralism.

Despite Dr. Garceau's tribute to the qualities of AMA members in the Introduction ("The AMA is a group of professional men par excellence . . . There is no group which has given more freely of itself" p. 11), the author sees the organization as beset with "very human and very political problems of internal government" (p. 12). He examines the organizational structure of the AMA and its affiliated societies, and concludes that the Association is in fact run by a small but well-organized "active minority." After a detailed examination of membership data (with numerous tables and charts), Dr. Garceau looks at how the AMA is actually governed, and concludes that the Association is run through maintenance of a complex balance between the national office and state and local societies, with the Chicago headquarters staffed by politically knowledgeable and clever activists (in particular, Dr. Morris Fishbein).

However, the author sees AMA unity as weakened by persistent tensions within the organization. On issues such as health insurance, there are major differences within the membership, and between state societies. "The AMA is in a sense the center of communication of a federal system, and as such it is faced with difficult problems of reconciliation" (p. 143). The author forecasts future external political difficulties for the organization, since "the political machinery and the political process have not provided adequate opportunities or at least adequate incentives for a thorough threshing out of group opinion" (pp. 152-153). Even a wide-open split cannot be ruled out. According to Dr. Garceau, the most important part of Association revival must be an acceptance of the legitimacy of political dissent by members over policy issues. Opponents must not be treated as heretics. To further this end, the author advocates the establishment of a formal political party system within the AMA.

In the final chapter, the author looks at the operations of the AMA within the national political arena. He concludes that "as a pressure group seeking control over public policy, the AMA is not, on balance, an unreasonably or dangerously powerful organization in the present political scene" (p. 167). Given its ideology of medical professionalism, an effective AMA can work for the public's interest as well as its own.

145. Ginzberg, Eli. *The Limits of Health Reform.* New York, NY: Basic Books, Inc., 1977.

This work is a continuation of Dr. Ginzberg's long-standing analysis of current U.S. health care policy, and possibilities for reform and improvement. On this occasion, the eminent scholar's work through the Conservation of Human Resources program at Columbia University was supported by grants from the Robert Wood Johnson Foundation and the U.S. Department of Labor.

The twelve-chapter text (with two hundred pages) is divided into three parts: "Framework", "Goals" and "Prospects for Reform". In Chapter Three ("The Postwar Experience"), Dr. Ginzberg briefly outlines American Medical Association opposition to national health insurance during the 1930-1950 period--opposition that successfully forestalled inaction of health insurance proposals advocated by the Roosevelt and Truman Administrations. In the same chapter, he also discusses AMA opposition to federal subsidies for medical schools and governmentally-sponsored expansion of medical school enrollments. However, the AMA was cooperated with the Medicare program "once it was assured that the new legislation would not be used to disturb existing relationships between physicians and their patients" (p. 31).

Within Ginzberg's narrative, there are also brief references to AMA opposition to HMOs (now lessened) and the admission of foreign medical graduates. The author concludes that AMA political power is now on the decline, given the rise of active specialty societies and falling AMA membership rolls. Nevertheless, the Association "retains considerable clout. It still is able to beat back most attempts that aim to alter the long-standing relations between physician and patient, to restrict the rights of the profession to practice according to its own goals, or to weaken its economic position" (p. 166).

146. Knause, Elliot A. *Power and Illness.* New York, NY: Elsevier, 1977.

In this three-part book Elliot Knause presents a general political social point of view which "shows how an essential resource (health) and an essential service (health care) are intimately involved with the political, economic, and social struggles of the present day" (Preface). Knause discusses a study of the context of health and health care and concludes the text with a suggestion that a National Health Service would better serve the American people. However, he does state his understanding that to change the system through reform there will be great political debate "with power, money, political organizations and ideologies" (p. 348).

Knause references the AMA quite extensively in this analysis of the political factors involved in the development of the U.S. Health

Care System. He discusses the AMA's opposition to Medicare, national health insurance and commercial blood bank centers, in its early conservative years. Also presented are the views that the AMA's leadership turned to liberal directions in the later 1960s, when they advocated the immigration of foreign doctors and assisted the federal government in establishing impossibly high standards for medical organizations. At one point, Knause even labels the AMA as a "monolithic organization"(p. 348). However, he points out that the organization returned to conservatism in the mid 1970s with policies oriented towards free enterprise in health care reform.

147. Knowles, John H., Editor. *Doing Better and Feeling Worse.* New York, NY: W. W. Norton and Company, 1977.

This volume is a collection of nineteen essays by a large and notable interdisciplinary group of scholars on an extremely wide range of health care system issues. To the extent that there is any integrative focus, it is on public policy options facing the United States in the Seventies and beyond. Within the readings, the American Medical Association receives very little attention. In the essay by Aaron Wildavsky ("Doing Better and Feeling Worse: The Political Pathology of Health Policy"), the author declares that "respect for the AMA has declined, its internal unity has diminished, and its congressional supporters have nearly vanished" (p. 114). On the other hand, in "Provider, Government, and Consumer", Merlin K. Duval emphasizes the historical power of the AMA in medical education and service provision. Eli Ginzberg ("Power Centers and Decision-Making Mechanisms") focuses on how institutional and technological changes within health care have led to the relative decline of traditional AMA power.

148. Kronenfeld, Jennie Jacobs and Marcia Lynn Whicker. *U.S. National Health Policy: An Analysis of the Federal Role.* New York, NY: Praeger Publishers, 1984.

As the title indicates, this book deals with the process and outcomes of health policy making at the federal level. The book's ten chapters (totaling slightly over two hundred text pages) deal with such issues as national health policies in the research, planning and service areas, federal health legislation, the economic factors of supply and demand, and equity.

In Chapter Four ("Politics and the Health Policy Process"), the authors briefly touch upon the role of the American Medical

Association in funding Political Action Committees (PACs), which funnel resources to favored congressional candidates during election campaigns. "Both national and state AMA-related health PACs were large contributors to favored candidates, together providing $5.6 million for candidates for the Ninety-Sixth Congress" (p. 66). Kronenfeld and Whicker also point out that MEDPAC, the AMA's coalition of PACs, is the largest single health-related interest group making campaign contributions. Concerning Medicare, the authors state that "the AMA has been active politically on any proposed changes that affect funding levels and reimbursement payments for physicians"(p. 67).

In Chapters Five ("Policy Process Outcomes") and Ten ("National Health Care Policy in the Future"), the authors mention that the AMA vigorously lobbies against undesirable policies. Examples cited include the Sheppard-Towner Act in the 1920s, and TEFRA legislation in the Eighties.

149. Lewis, Charles E., Rashi Fein and David Mechanic. *A Right to Health.* New York, NY: John Wiley & Sons, 1976.

This work, started with a grant from the Robert Wood Johnson Foundation, is subtitled "the problem of access to primary medical care". The authors (eminent and extensively published health policy scholars) take both conceptual and historical approaches in analyzing the problems that the U.S. has had in providing access to primary health care for all of its citizens. The book (over three hundred pages long, with nineteen chapters plus appendices) concludes with a section on policy options.

The authors principally look at the role of the American Medical Association in developing primary care in "Family Practice: the Primary Care Specialty" (Chapter 7). As they note, the AMA began efforts to develop recommendations for upgrading general practice in 1956. However, the twenty pilot family practice programs that were established as a result received inadequate support and interest, and ended in 1969. The AMA was more successful in gaining support for a family practice option when its Ad Hoc Committee on Education for Family Practice issued the Willard Report in 1966. The authors discuss the 1969 AMA recognition of the family practice specialty, and point out that the AMA and other organizations "have mounted promotional campaigns and extracurricular programs to involve students in primary care" (p. 82), and have subsequently surveyed medical schools to assess resulting changes in educational programs.

In Chapter Eight ("Efforts to Increase the Number of Physicians"), the authors briefly touch on the AMA policy shift in favor of increasing medical school enrollment in the early Sixties, including more (and more equitably distributed) primary care physicians. ". . . In 1973, the AMA president-elect included among organized medicine's priority goals an increase in primary care physicians and a better geographic distribution of health professionals, especially to deprived areas" (p. 93). They also describe the AMA physician surveys to ascertain the professional and geographic distribution of doctors.

150. Lewis, Irving J. and Cecil G. Sheps. *The Sick Citadel.* Cambridge, MA: Oelgeschlager, Gunn & Hain, Publishers, Inc., 1983.

This book, subtitled "The American Academic Medical Center and the Public Interest", is an investigation of the "role and power of the academic medical center and its fundamental dependence . . . on public policy" (p. xvii). The central contention of Irving J. Lewis and Cecil G. Sheps (professors at Yeshiva University and the University of North Carolina at Chapel Hill, respectively) is that the relationship between academic medical centers and government is inadequate for the demands of the 1980s. In an introduction, seven chapters and 250 pages, they outline the history of academic medical centers and their various roles in public policy, explain why things are not going well at present, and suggest how a new mission and a new model might improve things.

Chapter 1 ("The Evolution of Public Policy for Health Care") provides a general outline of government involvement in health care throughout U.S. history. For the purposes of this book, the key turning point came after World War II, when the Federal Government became heavily involved in subsidizing medical school enrollment and biomedical research. With such institutions as the National Institutes of Health (NIH) disbursing billions of dollars each year, the institutions that primarily benefited from such largesse--academic medical centers--became "big business". These policies may have worked all too well--the additional medical personnel and scientific advances obtained from the medical centers (along with such policy initiatives as Medicare and Medicaid) have played a part in igniting the cost inflation that currently plagues the U.S. health care system.

The authors describe academic medical centers, their roles in providing patient care and professional education, finances and governance in the next five chapters. Evolving more or less directly from the recommendations of the Flexner Report, the centers have become indispensable in both areas. Both federal and state governments have responded with increased funding. But as a consequence, these privileged centers have become alienated both from their host universities and the communities that surround them.

Within the centers themselves, components jostle each other for ever larger budgets. Departments and their physicians have become enamored with esoteric and specialized high technology medicine, and so relegate less glamorous concerns such as family practice and geriatrics to second-class status. With the high stakes involved, issues of governance become continually more important, and often bitterly disputed.

In Chapter 7, Lewis and Sheps survey the prevailing uncertainty regarding the proper role of the academic medical center, and strongly advocate a greater emphasis on service to the surrounding community. They also call for stronger executive control over the centers, and more sophisticated planning and budgeting systems. Finally, they conclude that "it is time to lay aside the Flexner Report as the only model for medical schools" (p. 230). Centers should become less universally concerned with research, and more attuned to the particular needs of their communities and regions. In this way, academic medical centers could more appropriately discharge their social responsibilities, and facilitate citizen participation in developing the modes of health care required for the Eighties and beyond.

151. Leyerle, Betty. *Moving and Shaking American Medicine.* Westport, CT: Greenwood Press, 1984.

The "movers and shakers" referred to in the title of Dr. Leyerle's book are corporations, and the "corporatization" of health care, in which previously autonomous health professionals and interest groups such as physicians and the American Medical Association are neutralized and brought under the firm control of business managers, is the subject of this work. Betty Leyerle is an Assistant Professor of Sociology and Human Services at Fort Lewis College. Her brief (seven chapters and 178 pages of text) book is part of the Contributions in Economics and Economic History series issued by Greenwood Press.

The subtitle of this book is "the structure of a socioeconomic transformation". Each of the seven chapters attempts to highlight a major aspect of this corporate-driven transformation. The "Introduction" (Chapter 1) provides an overview of the various ways in which "industry's strategy for change" (p. 18) involves altering both the means and ends of health care delivery. As the quoted term implies, Dr. Leyerle usually treats the corporate sector as a monolith, with common problems and attitudes with respect to health care issues. Chapter 2 focuses on "Reimbursement Policies of Third Party Payers," while Chapters 3 and 4 explore the operations of "Industrial Health Programs" and "Health Maintenance Organizations" respectively. The next two chapters look at "Corporate Roles in Health Care Planning" and "Provider Adaptations to Structural Pressures"--the opposing sides in conflicts over what the new health care system should look like, and who should control it. The "Conclusion" expresses doubt about the ultimate impact of this corporate transformation on health care costs, access and quality, but none regarding its inevitability.

At various points in the book, Dr. Leyerle outlines the power that physicians and the AMA have had in twentieth century American health care, and (until recently) the successful actions they have carried out to preserve it. Until the post-WWII era, the AMA opposed health insurance. The Association has also opposed the health systems agencies set up by the National Health Planning and Resources Development Act of 1974. In general, efforts to establish health services planning and rationalization--supported by the corporate sector and government--have been bitterly fought by physicians, who benefit from fragmented structure and authority. The supporters of planning, however, are steadily winning the day, as more detailed and elaborate controls on provider behavior are put in place.

Those physicians who are not being subjugated are being coopted; the AMA now favors physician participation on hospital boards, and many physicians are now becoming owner/administrators of facilities as well. Efforts to forestall corporate reform, such as the Voluntary Effort coalition that includes the AMA, are unlikely to stem this tide. Though AMA/physician influence may keep doctors' incomes up, the coming decades will see "the demise of the last of the free professions powerful enough to control their own work" (p. 178).

152. Marmor, Theodore R. and Jon B. Christianson. *Health Care Policy: A Political Economy Approach.* Beverly Hills, CA: Sage Publications, 1982.

This relatively brief (230 pages in nine chapters) work covers a variety of political and economic issues currently affecting the U.S. health care system. Several of the chapters are reprints from journal articles. Dr. Marmor is Chairman of the Center for Health Studies at Yale University, while Dr. Christianson is an Associate Professor in the areas of Public Policy, Planning, Administration and Economics at the University of Arizona in Tucson.

In "National Health Insurance" (Chapter 5), the authors analyze a variety of proposals for broadening health insurance coverage, including the Medicredit proposal of the American Medical Association, which would subsidize the purchase of private health insurance. They conclude that the AMA plan would increase the health purchasing power of low income groups, but would also reinforce practices that lead to cost inflation. In any event, adoption of

Medicredit "is unlikely as long as the Democrats control either the White House or Congress" (p. 113).

153. Marmor, Theodore R. *Political Analysis and American Medical Care.* New York, NY: Cambridge University Press, 1983.

As the author describes it, this work "is a collection of my essays on political analysis and the world of American medicine" (p. ix), primarily written in the Seventies. Dr. Marmor is a Professor and member of the Center for Health Studies at Yale University. These essays, most of which were co-authored with Dr. Marmor's students and faculty colleagues, reflect a concern for the impact of politics and ideology on health care. They also clearly reflect the authors' own broadly left-liberal ideology, with a particular emphasis on the unequal distribution of resources and power in the modern U.S. health care system.

The twelve essays in the book total about 250 pages of text. The essay subjects include (among others): medical inflation, consumer interests, health planning, welfare medicine, and the Canadian experience with national health insurance. The introductory essay, "Political Science and Health Services Administration", provides a general framework for analysis, while the Epilogue ("Medical Care and Pro Competitive Reform") offers Dr. Marmor's forecast for the Eighties and beyond.

In general, the essays in this book portray the American Medical Association as an influential interest group with an elitist and materialist orientation, but with limited power to impose or defend its interests. "The AMA clearly has influence on some policies, but their form is shaped more by an American ideological bias toward private control of medicine than by electoral pressure" (p. 14). The Association often succeeds through what the author terms "tacit bargaining", in which group interests are taken into account by policy makers without explicit negotiation (as in the case of Medicare program development).

With respect to the inaction of Medicare--often seen as a signal political defeat for the AMA--Marmor offers a dissenting opinion. The program's narrow focus on just one age group, the elderly, rather than the needs of the general public, "was a sop to AMA fears, and the exclusion of physician services benefits was a response to past AMA hysteria" (p. 138). Far from representing a defeat, Medicare took for granted, and left virtually undisturbed, the extensive privileges and power that physicians possessed within the U.S. health care system. The program's inaction therefore confirmed more than challenged the power of the AMA and the physician profession.

In the Epilogue, Dr. Marmor contends that pro competitive policy will in fact become pro-business, anti-regulatory policy-- an effort to reduce corporate and government expenditures without significantly altering the distribution of medical power and resources within the U.S. The AMA may indeed lose influence as the monopolistic practices of physicians are eroded by antitrust actions (the removal of the AMA ban on physician advertising, for example). But "pro competitive arguments will politically rationalize the attack on contemporary health regulations without fundamentally reforming the industry" (p. xvi). One set of elites (corporate managers) will replace another (physicians and the AMA) at the top of the health care system, but true equality in American health care will be just as distant as before.

154. Poen, Monte M. *Harry S Truman Versus the Medical Lobby*. Columbia, MO: University of Missouri Press, 1979.

Originally a doctoral dissertation, this work explores the conflicts between President Harry S Truman and "the medical lobby" (in particular, the American Medical Association) over Truman's proposals for health care reform, especially national health insurance. The author also analyzes the linkages between Truman's "failure" and President Lyndon Johnson's success in getting Medicare enacted in 1965. The text is detailed but concise (230 pages in nine chapters), and is accompanied by an extensive bibliography listing primary and secondary sources.

The first two chapters provide a summary of events before Truman's accession to the Presidency, including the background debate over health insurance from 1915 - 1941, and President Franklin Roosevelt's concerns with national health policy. The AMA here, as throughout the book, is portrayed as a powerful and skillful foe of efforts to establish any system of national health care. The AMA's task of opposition was relatively easy in the Twenties, with little national reform spirit existing. With the election of Roosevelt and the rise of the New Deal in the 1930s, pro-health insurance efforts increased, but Congressional support (as symbolized by the Wagner Bill) was dissipated by Presidential reluctance to act in the face of strong AMA opposition, and the Chief Executive's gradual preoccupation with foreign affairs as World War II began.

AMA concerns rose again during and after the war, since the conflict inevitably drew the Federal Government further into the health care sector. Led by Morris Fishbein, the Association furiously (and successfully) lobbied Congress against the Wagner- Murray-Dingell bill for health insurance. FDR's plans to more strongly push for the measure were ended with his death in 1945.

Incoming President Harry Truman was an unknown quantity, but he soon turned out to be a more open and combative advocate of national health insurance than his predecessor. Chapters 3 - 6 of the book outline Truman's efforts to get a program through Congress. The AMA moderated its stance to the extent of supporting the Hill-Burton Hospital Construction Act of 1946, but its advocacy of a voluntary sickness insurance system fell far short of what Truman wanted. A coalition including the AMA, the American Hospital Association, Catholic and Protestant hospital groups, the American Bar Association and the U.S. Chamber of Commerce stopped all of the attempts at significant health service reform during the 1946 - 1949 period, aided by the brilliant Whitaker-Baxter public relations campaign. However, in the author's view, Truman's defeats did in fact pave the way for future victories for health insurance supporters with the passage of Medicare (Chapter 7).

Poen suggests in Chapters 8 and 9 that the AMA, increasingly inflexible in tactics and doctrine, steadily lost ground as growing governmental involvement in health care "contributed to a widening of the ideological gulf separating the free-enterprise-oriented private practitioner, as represented by the AMA, from those who depended upon public funding: the medical educators, researchers and hospital employees" (p. 215).

155. Sidel, Victor W., and Sidel, Ruth. *A Healthy State*. New York, NY: Pantheon Books, 1983.

The book, originally issued in 1977 and significantly updated for its 1983 edition, provides "an international perspective on the crisis in United States medical care" (the subtitle). Victor W. Sidel is Chairperson of the Department of Social Medicine at Montefiore Medical Center and Professor of Community Health at the Albert Einstein College of Medicine in New York City. Ruth Sidel is a Professor of Sociology at Hunter College, City University of New York. In seven chapters spanning almost 350 pages, the authors look at the U.S. health care system, compare it to medical delivery in Sweden, Great Britain, the Soviet Union, and the People's Republic of China (each described in a separate chapter), and, based upon their investigation, provide proposals for major reform in America's health policy. Firmly situated on the political left, Victor and Ruth Sidel are clear in their preferences for a national health services system in the U.S.

Though not providing a detailed analysis, the authors do indict the American Medical Association as a basically reactionary organization that obstructs necessary progress in service delivery. At one point, the

AMA is criticized for doing away with "much of the role of women in medicine in the United States" (p. 228). The authors admit that there was a "liberal" strain in the AMA's policy prescriptions in the early decades of the 20th Century. But "in the early 1920's, the AMA was taken over by a group of private practitioners . . . and the organization began to function as a much more clearly defined special-interest group" (p. 237) with reactionary objectives. The AMA has contributed to the establishment of a pernicious and inequitable two-tier health care system within the U.S. Consequently, progressive health care reform will require, among other things, the reduction of AMA political and social influence.

156. Sidel, Victor W. and Sidel, Ruth., Editors. *Reforming Medicine.* New York, NY: Pantheon Books, 1984.

This reader (subtitled "lessons of the last quarter century") provides a variety of policy-oriented perspectives in five parts (and approximately 280 pages): "health care institutions", "services for special groups", "health workers", "control of health care". The editors, as well as most of the authors, are members of the political left, and dedicated to reforming the current American health care system. While they take time to celebrate the successes of the Sixties and Seventies, they nevertheless see much that remains to be done, and many efforts that need to be redirected.

The general attitude of the authors toward the American Medical Association is one of hostility. The AMA is portrayed as a powerful and effective interest group for the wealthy (physicians and others), dedicated to promoting privilege and inequality as integral characteristics of capitalist medicine.

157. Stevens, Robert and Rosemary Stevens. *Welfare Medicine in America.* New York, NY: The Free Press, 1974.

This book is a study of the Medicaid Program, which in 1973 provided health care for 23 million Americans. The Stevenses describe the social-welfare program extensively in this four part volume. Beginning with the "Coming of Medicaid" and spanning to what they call "Benign Neglect," the authors study the historical process which lead to the structure and administration of Medicaid. They examine what happened once the legislation was enacted, how the States interpreted their individual roles in the program, and the final efforts of the program administrator and the governmental legislators to address the problems of the Medicaid Program.

In reference to the AMA, the Stevenses spoke of the Association's decision concerning the issue of compulsory health insurance in the late fifties and early sixties. They illustrate the effectiveness of the lobbying powers of the AMA to running interference with respect to national health insurance. The AMA endorsed a national health insurance plan but one that was based on a system of tax credits called Medicredit.

Stevens did discuss the AMA's push for professional standard review organizations. He also presented that by 1974 the AMA had lost most of its influence of the 1960's. Again, the Stevenses related very little of the AMA to this study of the Medicaid Program.

158. Stevens, Rosemary. *In Sickness and in Wealth.* New York, NY: Basic Books, Inc., 1989.

What are the proper relationships between hospitals and physicians? To what extent can U.S. hospitals be run like "businesses"—corporate enterprises—while remaining true to their essential clinical mission? This are major issues in Rosemary Stevens' survey of "American Hospitals in the Twentieth Century" (the subtitle of the book). Dr. Stevens is Professor and Chairman of the Department of History and Sociology of Science at the University of Pennsylvania. In the book, the author tries to show how a lack of national consensus over the answers to these questions has led the hospital industry to its state of uncertainty in the 1990s.

The text itself consists of thirteen chapters, and is over four hundred pages long, including an extensive "notes" section at the end. In Chapter 3 ("A National Enterprise: Setting Basic Rules"), Dr. Stevens points out that hospital standardization was an important and logical consequence of the doctors' reform movement led by the American Medical Association. "The American Medical Association's policies . . . also defined the hospital as the workshop of a responsible profession of practitioners. In so doing, standardization upheld the organizational separation of hospitals and physicians . . . and supported private practice" (p. 52). The author also provides a section in the chapter on the Flexner Report and its impact upon medical education.

In the 1920's, the AMA vigorously supported hospital expansion and building programs, particularly in rural areas. "AMA policy was simply that every doctor should have a hospital within his or her local territory. . . . The AMA and its constituent societies . . . were thus more interested in the number of hospitals than in the overall supply of beds" (p. 119). This support, however, did not apply to veterans' hospitals, which the AMA bitterly opposed. The fact that they were governmentally run was a primary factor in this stance. "The AMA rose in strength in the 1920s, using federal programs as a rallying cry to consolidate its role as the constituency of the average, local private practitioner" (p. 128). Thus began the AMA campaign against "socialized medicine".

In the Thirties, voluntary hospitals and physicians moved closer together, bound by opposition to schemes for more nationalized health care. "State and national hospital associations, growing as articulators of the voluntary ideal, took care not to offend the American Medical Association and its state and local affiliates, and not to confront private practitioners by ruthless competition with them" (p. 150). Morris Fishbein, Editor of JAMA, argued for an alliance between hospitals and physicians to oppose group practice and government involvement in health care. On the other hand, the AMA was willing to endorse the concept of voluntary hospital insurance, as long as it required fee-for- service doctors to provide care. The success of Blue Cross, for example, came from the mutually supportive ties it fostered between "the mainline ideologies of both voluntary hospitals and the medical profession, thus building the reputation of the AHA and tying it more closely to the American Medical Association" (p. 190).

After the Second World War, the hospital/physician alliance successfully labored to gain large federal subsidies through inaction of the Hill-Burton Act. By the Fifties, however, strains were appearing in the coalition, with hospitals pushing for more authority over physician practices within their facilities. The notion of "the corporate practice of medicine" became widely debated, and the AMA became suspicious of the growing power of the Joint Commission on Accreditation of Hospitals to set standards of hospital performance.

By the late Sixties, health care cost containment had moved to the fore as an issue, and the interests of physicians and hospitals diverged even further. The adoption of the Medicare prospective payment system forced hospitals to closely monitor physician behavior, and AMA surveys were showing that physicians felt that their very status as independent professionals was being threatened.

159. Strickland, Stephen P. *U.S. Health Care: What's Wrong and What's Right.* New York, NY: Universe Books, 1972.

This short (six chapters and 109 text pages) book provides a survey of the state of the U.S. health care system in the early Seventies. Topics covered include the federal government's role in health care, the nature of the system's "crisis" and proposed solutions, and changes taking place within the medical profession. Data from a variety of health policymaker and practitioner surveys conducted by Potomac Associates are analyzed as well. In the first part of the book, the author frequently refers to the influence of the American Medical Association on national health policy. He notes the AMA's gradual shift toward acceptance of a public responsibility for providing health care for all citizens, and the need for more physicians to carry out this responsibility. In a section of Chapter III entitled "Participants in the Policy Process", it is reported that "citizens put greater confidence and trust in 'organizations of doctors' such as the American Medical Association than in any other single group identified as a potential contributor to the development of new federal health legislation" (p. 55). Physicians, particularly solo general practitioners, place greater trust in the AMA than other health professional groups.

In Chapter IV ("Evaluation of Proposed Solutions") Strickland describes the AMA's Medicredit proposal for health insurance, as well as the split between office-based, fee-for-service general practitioners (generally opposed) and their hospital-based, specialized and/or salaried counterparts (generally supportive) over the desirability of national health insurance. A similar split within the AMA ranks can be found over the issue of HMO development.

160. Stroman, Duane F. *The Medical Establishment and Social Responsibility*. Port Washington, NY: Kennikat Press, 1976.

To what extent is the physician profession responsible for the ills that currently beset the U.S. health care system? According to Duane F. Stroman, an Associate Professor of Sociology at Juniata College in Huntingdon, PA, doctors deserve a great deal of blame for the cost, quality and access shortcomings in U.S. health care. Since the turn of the century, physicians have dominated the service delivery and regulatory institutions of American medicine, but have failed to develop the modern management expertise that is required. In this short and somewhat dated book (under two hundred pages, including seven chapters, an appendix and bibliography), Stroman outlines the range of deficiencies in the U.S. health delivery system, links them to the excessive professional autonomy and dominance of physicians, and suggests how the nation might move "toward a social ethic for health care" (p. 140). In the first four chapters, Stroman looks at the present state of health care, and how social and professional changes are leading to growing inadequacies in service planning and delivery.

Despite its great potential, American health care is all too often unequally distributed, and the payment structure is haphazard and inefficient. The quality of care is often substandard, and features an impersonality that must be deemed unacceptable. At the same time, the application of new technologies and changing population needs further unsettle the health industry. Reflecting these developments, new health professions have risen, each demanding respect and a share of the decision-making power and responsibility. Consumers of health services are also becoming more sophisticated, and are calling for greater professional accountability and regulation.

According to the author, the consequence of all this is pervasive disarray, with health professionals and institutions unable to adequately respond to these new challenges. "Our health care system . . . has been described as a cottage industry in an age of conglomerates, while physicians are described as pushcart vendors in an age of supermarkets" (p. 59). Health services planning and coordination are too crude to meet the new requirements, so the U.S. has a "huge gap between science and service" (p. 94). In Chapter 4, Stroman traces these problems to physician dominance and independence, excessive private entrepreneurship, an overemphasis on scientific achievement, and a systemwide anti-bureaucratic and anti-planning orientation.

Professional dominance, responsibility and self-regulation are analyzed in detail by the author in the next two chapters. Though it is not without its good points, the "ideology of organized medicine" leads to the self-aggrandizement of the physician profession at the expense of consumers, other health care professionals, and the nation as a whole. After looking at licensure, peer review and other mechanisms, Stroman concludes that "the wide gulf between the promise and the reality of self-regulation does not justify the medical profession's nearly unfettered control of its own operations" (p. 139).

In the final chapter ("Toward a Social Ethic for Health Care"), the author outlines his own prescriptions for reform. In general, they involve greater public participation in and governmental control over health services provision. A federal health board should be established to coordinate and rationalize federal and voluntary health programs and activities. The board would also supervise the development of a system of regional and national health planning, and a program of national health insurance. Stroman suggests that this board should be "so constituted that it is not dominated by elitist medical interests but is focused on the centrality of patient needs which can be voiced by means of lay representation" (p. 154). Physician reimbursement, professional licensure and quality assurance systems also need to be upgraded and nationally standardized.

161. Taylor, Lloyd C., Jr. *The Medical Profession and Social Reform, 1885-1945*. New York, NY: St. Martin's Press, 1974.

As the title indicates, this book is an historical account of the relationship between the physician profession and various issues of "social reform" that were important during the same period. The author, Lloyd C. Taylor, Jr., is a professor at Texas A & M University. The text itself is concise (163 pages), and divided into nine chapters that cover such topics as industrial and social reform, the movement for public health, and the impact of the world wars on "social medicine".

In Chapter 6 ("World War I: The War for Public Health"), Dr. Taylor notes that the post-war movement for health insurance and group medicine was completely rejected by the AMA on the grounds that both developments would destroy the doctor-patient relationship, curb freedom of choice for both actors, and reduce medical practice to an assembly-line process. The author also links this opposition to the fact that these reforms would lead to more specialist training and utilization, while most AMA members were general practitioners. It was therefore in the professional self-interest of the AMA to oppose these reforms.

"The 1920s and the Fate of Social Medicine" (Chapter 7) covers the activities of Arthur B. Emmons II and the Harvard Mercantile Health Work. His advocacy of contract medicine was strongly criticized by many AMA members, who felt it would undermine the economic status and security of most doctors. During the same time period, the AMA attacked the proposed Sheppard-Towner Act for the Protection of Maternity and Infancy, since it would have entailed federal government financial support for public health. The Act was passed, but continual AMA opposition facilitated its nullification in 1929. Since many subsequent reform proposals were identified with progressive and "radical" individuals such as Alice Hamilton, Hugh Cabot and Martha Eliot, the AMA became more conservative in response.

This political tendency continued in the Thirties (Chapter 8, "The New Deal in Medicine"), with AMA attacks on the work of the Committee on the Costs of Medical Care (CCMC). Once again, the AMA criticized a social reform proposal on the grounds that it would destroy the all-important system of private practice, and institute socialism via contract medicine. AMA opposition also ensured that the Social Security Act of 1935 would largely ignore medical considerations. Despite these developments, social reformers (with the low-key support of the Roosevelt Administration) continued to push for medical reform, particularly with respect to government subsidies. Criticism of the AMA's hostility to reform proposals steadily mounted.

The Forties constituted an "encore for social medicine" (Chapter 9), with vigorous (though unsuccessful) attempts to enact the National Health Act. The dislocations caused by World War II finally enabled the Federal Government to involve itself financially with health services through the First Deficiency Appropriation Act for emergency maternal and child care. Despite AMA opposition to this and the subsequent Wagner-Murray-Dingell bill for national health care, the Federal Government had arrived as a permanent participant in the provision of health services.

162. Weeks, Lewis E. and Howard J Berman. *Shapers of American Health Policy: An Oral History.* Ann Arbor, MI: Health Administration Press, 1985.

This detailed historical work includes the fruits of over forty oral histories of influential figures in U.S. health policy making in the last fifty years, including such luminaries as Odin W. Anderson, Wilbur J. Cohen, Gary L. Filerman and Wilbur D. Mills. Lewis Weeks heads the oral history project, which is housed in the Library of the American Hospital Association. Howard J. Berman is President of Blue Cross and Blue Shield of Rochester, New York. The text is divided into four parts ("Cornerstones", "Blue Cross: An Evolving Social Movement", "The Emergence of a Profession", and "A Look Backward"), covering approximately 260 pages.

Since the book covers U.S. health policy during the Twentieth Century, it (and the oral histories) frequently refer to the American Medical Association. Two of the staff members of the Committee on the Costs of Medical Care (CCMC), I. S. Falk and C. Rufus Rorem, provide an inside account of the committee's confrontation with the AMA over the concepts of health planning and health maintenance organizations. Falk went on to work for the Committee on Economic Security in the Roosevelt Administration, and recounts the AMA's lobbying activities against inclusion of health insurance in the Social Security Act. Public health and material, child health and welfare concerns did survive in Titles V and VI of the Act.

Others discussing the impact of the AMA include Wilbur Cohen (who discusses Association opposition to health insurance proposals by the Kennedy Administration, and the final compromises with the AMA over Medicare), George Bugbee (who talks about the difficulties encountered in getting the American Hospital Association out from under the shadow of the AMA), and Maurice J. Norby (who covers the interactions between the AMA and the AHA over the establishment of what would become the JCAH).

In the final chapter ("Five Decades of Change"), the authors provide a broad summary of policy events, and frequently refer to the AMA's influence. In particular, the role of AMA opposition to the proposed National Health Bill in 1939, and various health insurance proposals during the Truman, Kennedy and Johnson Administrations are described. They conclude with the successful passage of Medicare and Medicaid in 1965.

163. Yaggy, Duncan and Patricia Hodgson, Editors. *Physicians and Hospitals*. Durham, NC: Duke University Press, 1985.

This is a collection of presentations and responses that took place at the Ninth Private Sector Conference on health care in Durham, North Carolina. Sponsored by the Duke Endowment, the conference attracted many nationally prominent physicians, hospital administrators and health services scholars to discuss the sometimes strained relationships between American hospitals and the doctors working within them. American Medical Association participants included Joseph F. Boyle (President-Elect), Alan Nelson (Trustee) and James H. Sammons (Executive Vice President).

All three AMA participants have commentaries in the text. James Sammons is critical of the newly-enacted Medical Prospective Payment system, suggesting that it will strain the hospital-physician relationship and interfere with physicians' medical judgments. With respect to physician supply, he states that "it is the AMA's often-stated point of view that the decision about the size of medical school classes rests precisely where it belongs: in the hands of the faculties of the universities with which these schools are associated" (p. 55).

Joseph Boyle makes a presentation entitled "Doctors Create a Corporation to Deal with a Hospital." Although he states that "the AMA believes hospital medical staffs do have a right to protect their interests, so we are encouraging them to arrange for their own legal counsels" (p. 91), he is critical of increasing legalism within health care. He concludes that greater cooperation between hospitals, their administrators, and physicians will be more fruitful in the long run.

Making one of the concluding summaries of the conference, Alan Nelson is skeptical of the utility of competition between physicians and hospitals, and suspicious of increasing federal government cost containment efforts. He also vigorously opposes any efforts to directly involve physicians in health care rationing to patients, and predicts that rationing pressures will further irritate the hospital-physician relationship.

In the concluding discussion, there is debate regarding the unwillingness of the AMA to take a more explicit position regarding the desirable physician supply for the United States. In response to criticism on this issue by Eli Ginzberg, James Sammons admits that "maybe the AMA does need to re-address the question of physician manpower, but I have the feeling that, if we re-address it and we say anything, we would probably say basically what I've just said. We would probably not decide to markedly reduce admissions and enrollments in the United States" (p. 185). David Ottensmeyer calls for physicians and the AMA to carefully reexamine the benefits and liabilities of the fee-for-service system.

(B) Articles

164. "AMA to Forge a National Health Policy." *Medical World News* (July 5, 1982): 8-15.

This article accounts the major issues acted upon by the AMA's annual convention in 1982. Foremost was the Association's decision to approve a two-year $3 million effort to set medical care priorities and cooperate with other health groups in forging a national health policy. The AMA has elected to participate as a key leader rather than let federal and state health planners fill a void of inaction. Other issues included concern for a doctor surplus, foreign medical schools, specialization versus general practice, and federal support for HMOs.

165. Appelbaum, Alan L. and Mary A. Grayson. "AMA Withdraws from LCCME, Modifies Stand on Chiropractors as Delegates Meet in Chicago." *Hospitals* 53(16) (August 16, 1979): 17-20.

This article provides an excellent example of policy deliberations in AMA's House of Delegates in the late 1970s. The AMA in 1979 was facing monthly legal fees of approximately $100,000 to defend against matters such as lawsuits by chiropractors and the Federal Trade Commission; in response, the Association elected to soften its language, dropping references to chiropractors as a "nonscientific cult", while calling attention to the limitations of chiropractic treatment. The delegates furthermore announced the AMA would withdraw from the Liaison Committee on Continuing Medical Education (LCCME) in concern that the Committee's current proposal to create state or regional entities would lessen the influence of state medical associations in the accreditation process. The authors additionally summarize the delegates' concerns regarding declining AMA membership, dues increases, medical ethics, and physician interests in the Joint Commission on Accreditation of Hospitals. The article concludes with AMA's continued resistance to compulsory national health insurance proposals.

166. Boyle, Joseph F. "The Health Policy Agenda (HPA) for the American People." *Journal of American Medical Association* 249 (15) (April 15, 1983): 2073.

This brief article summarizes the background and purpose of AMA's 1982 initiative to create a conceptual and philosophical frame to guide U.S. health policy development for the next five to ten years. The Association dedicated approximately $3.5 million and manpower to coordinate the efforts of over 150 health care organizations. HPA will provide a set of principles and policy on specific issues that provide a common basis for working social, economic, scientific, educational, and political issues.

167. Boyle, Joseph F. "The Challenges of Health Care in America, On the Side of the Patient." *Vital Speeches* LI (14) (May 1, 1985): 2073.

Dr. Boyle, as AMA President, begins this address with a summary of government intervention in health care, basic statistics on the magnitude of U.S. health care today, and a summary of great progress in medicine made in the last three decades. The author then centers on "This decade's crisis cost." Dr. Boyle accounts for measures physicians and hospitals have taken to contain costs, while costs for liability insurance has skyrocketed. Dr. Boyle then provides what AMA is doing to address these challenges, such as participation with 150 organizations to develop a Health Policy Agenda for the American People. The author makes it clear that AMA policy continues to promise that the health and welfare of patients shall be the first consideration, not allowing economics, politics, race, religion, or any other circumstances to take preference.

168. Bronson, Gail. "Relations Between Physicians and Chiropractors Are a Hot Issue at Medical Association Meeting." *The Wall Street Journal* (December 5, 1978): 48.

This article reflects the continued opposition between allopathic doctors and chiropractors. In May 1977, a Pennsylvania chiropractor filed a class-action suit against a hospital and various medical groups with restraint of trade for denying him and his patients diagnostic services. In a preliminary settlement of the suit, AMA trustees have agreed that physicians can accept patients also under a chiropractor's care and that hospitals, radiologists, and pathologists may provide diagnostic services to the same. The court actions immediately prompted a counterattack by angry doctors who believe this submission by AMA will promote the practice of unscientific medicine.

169. Chapman-Cliburn, Greg. "AMA Addresses Medical Staff Self-Governance." *Hospitals* (January 20, 1988): 84-85.

This short article provides examples of AMA's concern for medical staff self-governance, the role of medical directors, relationships between the medical staff and governing body and similar matters. With new regulations on hospital governance being considered by New York State, the AMA's Hospital Medical Staff Section recommended policy resolutions to the House of Delegates for their work with state medical societies regarding such legislation.

170. Day, Barbara and Howard Waitzkin. "The Medical Profession and Nuclear War." *Journal of American Medical Association* 254 (1985): 644-651.

This article provides a social history of the medical profession's response to federal civil defense programs and the dangers of nuclear war. The authors point out that the AMA and AHA have both generally supported civil defense measures since 1947. Only recently has the AMA called on state and local affiliates to educate doctors and the public about nuclear war and its medical consequences. This article also documents the efforts of several anti-nuclear war physician associations including Physicians for Social Responsibility and International Physicians for the Prevention of Nuclear War. These groups have made a significant impact with public information programs providing details on the nature and magnitude of destruction from nuclear war. The authors underline the changes in U.S. civil defense policy and anti-war activism as nuclear weapons and strategy change and the cold war waxes and wanes.

171. Deets, Horace B. "Health Care for a Caring America." *Vital Speeches* LV(20) (August 1, 1989): 636-637.

The speaker, as Executive Director of the American Association of Retired Persons (AARP), presents his Association's advocacy for immediate reform of the U.S. health care system. Deets faults the current system for ignoring preventive medicine, having 37 million uninsured Americans, insurance costs, which are too burdensome for business, and ineffective quality control and waste of resources. Deets says "we don't want a system in which government provides medical care and runs the medical profession. But government can and should establish guidelines, set standards, oversee quality of care and provide an overall funding mechanism, while individuals should remain free to choose their own doctors and hospitals." The author concludes with positive endorsement of initiatives by the National Leadership Commission on Health Care, the Washington Business Group on Health and Senator Kennedy's bill to extend coverage for uninsured Americans.

172. Demkovich, Linda E. "AMA, Government Officials Skeptical of 'Convenience Medicine' Facilities." *National Journal* (November 26, 1983): 2470-2473.

This article discusses the rapid growth of urgent care facilities (a.k.a. freestanding emergency centers and convenience medicine facilities), and the response of organized medicine, state and federal government. These facilities, not financially or physically connected with hospitals, typically offer lower charges and longer operating hours, and do not require appointments. While their growth has not competed against hospital emergency rooms, they very likely do compete with care provided in private physician offices. In 1983, the AMA was suggesting guidelines for state licensing of the facilities. The AMA reportedly was concerned about the freestanding emergency center association, and in response asked the Federal Trade Commission to act against the AMA's attempted restraint of trade.

Finally, local and state planning authorities were also considering imposing the requirement for convenience medicine facilities to receive certificates of need before expanding or renovating -- just as hospitals do. As intense competition for patients increases, the impact of convenience medicine should continue.

173. Ehrenreich, Barbara and John Ehrenreich. "Health Care and Social Control." *Social Policy* (May/June 1974): 26-40.

The authors are professors in the Health Sciences (Barbara) and American Studies (John) Departments at the State University of New York, Old Westbury. The article provides a unique treatment of the social control functions of the U.S. medical system. The Ehrenreichs account for changes in U.S. medicine and its impact on social control from the late 19th century to the present. The authors categorize types of medical social control as 1) Disciplinary control rising from Exclusionary forces that discourages the poor from getting sick and missing work, and 2) Co-operative control rising from expansionary medicine that encourages treatment of the middle and upper class in areas such as preventive care, and family planning. The authors trace the vast expansion of the medical system since 1930 with new technology, insurance coverage, and a growing dependency and desire of our population to receive the best possible care for more and more areas of treatment.

At the same time, the authors trace the rapid rise in status and class position of doctors. The Ehrenreichs combine these changes in our medical system and claim that doctors, through their ultimate authoritarian position over patients, often communicate ideological and moral messages which promote the position of the wealthy, the dominance of males, and their solutions on issues regarding sex, drugs, and alcohol. The article warns that physicians almost autonomously all call the shots on many social problems such as management of reproduction and death -- problems and solutions, for which the general public must assume responsibility.

174. Elliott, John. "Osteopaths Relax Membership Policy." *American Medical News* (August 3/10 1979): 19.

This very brief article records an event indicative of the infighting within organized medicine and illustrates the impact of federal regulators. Fearing anti-trust action by the Federal Trade Commission (FTC) similar to that in 1979 by the FTC against the AMA, the American Osteopathic Association (AOA), voted to allow its members to join the AMA and specialty societies outside the osteopathic profession. In addition, osteopaths are no longer required to hold membership in the AOA in order to serve on the professional staff of any osteopathic hospital. This major policy change additionally helps osteopaths receive malpractice insurance, third party reimbursement, specialty training, and continuing education through AMA-affiliated programs. The AOA still criticizes the AMA for trying to eliminate the osteopathic profession and intends to remain separate from allopathic medicine.

175. Foreman, Julie. "AMA Unveils Plan to Strengthen U.S. Health Care System." *Archives of Ophthalmology* 108 (May 1990): 649.

This article provides an excellent, one-page summary of AMA's "Health Access America" Plan to correct problems with the U.S. health care system. The plan is seen as a first step by AMA to bring over 150 lay players together to reach a consensus on needed action. AMA seeks to preserve the strengths of our present system (freedom of choice by patients regarding where and who provides them care, technological advances, strong research, superlative medical education and individualized patient care). Moreover, Health Access America would provide affordable coverage to all Americans, regardless of income. Foreman's article details the plan's sixteen main points.

176. Griffith, Hurdis. "Physician Payment Reform: Implications For Nurses." *Nursing Economics* 7 (4) (July-August 1989): 231-233.

This article describes the battle between the AMA and Congress over comprehensive physician payment reforms designed to lower Medicare costs. In the fall of 1987, it was announced that Medicare beneficiaries would face a 38.5% increase in Medicare premiums. Several Congressmen responded with charges that escalating Medicare payments to physicians increased at a rate twice the gross national product growth. In 1988, the Congressional Physician Payment Review Commission recommended a fee schedule for physician payment based on a resource-based relative value scale (RBRVS). The fee schedule would be determined by the cost of resources used to provide the service. Griffith's article calls on nurses to get involved because payment reforms will apply to them as well as physicians.

177. Hanley, Richard J. "Cost Containment of Health Care - The Responsibility of Employees and Doctors." *Vital Speeches* LI (3) (November 15, 1984): 74-77.

The speaker, as Vice President of Health Care Policy and Programs, Owens, Illinois, Inc., challenges all participants in the health care system to do a better job at cost containment. Hanley describes how his major corporation took aggressive cost containment action with great success. Owens redesigned their health benefit plans, increasing deductibles and employee contributions. They made a second opinion mandatory for certain surgical practices. Owens increased coverage for outpatient options and decreased those for inpatient treatment of the same illness. The Corporation's educational programs increased employee understanding of their options and fostered preventive care. Owens supports managed care programs, utilization reviews and legislative surveillance. Their senior management personally backs the entire cost containment strategy.

The speaker concludes by calling on doctors to support a nine-point cost containment program through cutting excess provider capacity, utilization review, serving more patients outside expensive delivery environments, participating in managed care programs, actively educating patients as to choices of care and the need for healthy lifestyles, and insisting on efficiency in hospitals.

178. Hawkins, Theron C. "Should the Texas Medical Association (TMA) Unify? "No!" *Texas Medicine* 85 (April 1989): 6-7.

The author, as member of the Texas Medical Association (TMA) House of Delegates, makes a case for not requiring doctors to join AMA as well as state and local medical societies. In 1989, about 60% of TMA members belonged to the AMA. Hawkins claims "AMA has a long history of opposing bad government health programs and then compromising away principles and ending up with things like Medicare, PSRO, PRO activities, the fee freeze, and low Medicaid reimbursements." The author says efforts to make "unified membership" mandatory will reduce TMA membership in local county societies.

179. Holahan, John; Moon, Marilyn; Welch, William Pete; and Zuckerman, Stephen. "An American Approach to Health System Reform." *Journal of the American Medical Association* 265 (19) (May 15, 1991): 2537-2540.

This article provides AMA's proposal for national health insurance as an alternative to other plans like the U.S. Government's proposal by the Pepper Commission. The AMA recognizes several major problems with the current U.S. health care system: There are over 32 million Americans at any one time with no coverage; during a recent 28-month period, 63 million Americans were lacking health insurance; the already very high costs of health care are increasing at least 4% per year above inflation; and finally, the current system is too complex administratively. The AMA proposal builds on many of the ideas proposed by the March 1990 Pepper Commission and portions of the Canadian system.

There are six principal measures of the AMA plan: 1) It would cover everyone through Medicare, employer-based coverage, state public programs (replacing Medicaid); 2) Employer-based and public programs would provide a standard minimum package of benefits and contain laws on maximum cost-sharing; 3) Employers and/or insurance companies would continue to administer private programs. The states would administer public programs; 4) The states would be required to control costs of public programs to preclude increases above GNP growth; 5) Employers would have the option of paying into a public plan or providing their own coverage; and the poor and unemployed would be subsidized; and 6) insurance companies would continue to underwrite, therefore stay in business, while tax increases would be somewhat limited by employer-based coverage. The AMA admits that their proposal would not be without problems. For example, small business profitability could be endangered, some states might not be capable of performing their portion, and taxes would unquestionably increase at federal and state levels.

180. Holden, Constance. "Doctors Must Put Patients First, Says Editor." *Science* 210 (November 7, 1980): 612-613.

This brief article cites an appeal by Arnold S. Relman, editor of the New England Journal of Medicine, to doctors to avoid having any financial association with the private health services market. Relman furthermore asks doctors not to hold stock in pharmaceutical or medical supply and equipment corporations. Relman sees a clear conflict of interest with the doctor serving as the purchasing agent for the patient, while the for-profit hospital or diagnostic center is the seller, and the public pays the major share of the bill. The author notes that "the AMA, as might be expected, does not see any virtue in Relman's views." The association says their policy and code of ethics are already adequate in their guidance, and that "there is no evidence of significant abuse by doctors of their combined roles as healers and businessmen."

181. Horner, David B. "The Battle for Control of Health Care." *Vital Speeches* LI(3) (November 15): 93-96.

The author, as President of the California Medical Association, provides a meaty, short address on the causes of rising health costs and expenditures and the government business and hospital management response to them. Horner cautions against overreliance on profit making health care systems which do not, in his opinion, have the patient's care as number one priority. The author warns that both government and business response now promote the rationing of health care and the use of the least costly practices and methods, and thereby do not have the patient's best interest at heart. He concludes with the statement that only the physician is looking out for the interest of the patient.

182. Hanlon, C. Rollins. "Shattuck Lecture - The Physician and Organized Medicine." *The New England Journal of Medicine* 284 (13) (May 20, 1971): 1131-1134.

Dr. Hanlon calls on doctors to be more than a solitary practitioner concerned about one-to-one relation with patients. Hanlon advocates joining political coalitions within organized medicine, expanding the physician's societal role and self-regulating the profession so that the public will respect organized medicine and support its continued independence. The author addresses the major changes in practicing health care, such as federal funding of medical research, rising expectations of the patient consumer, third-party payments, and federal legislation such as Medicare and Medicaid. Hanlon says that organized medicine must acknowledge it cannot provide the best possible medical care to everyone now. Therefore, it must work within a concept of a national health policy which determines where our limited resources should be allocated. Developing that policy is beyond the control of the AMA, AAMC and other specialty groups, and must be addressed by coalitions of health care providers, patient consumers, and government.

183. Kahn, Henry S. and Peter Orris. "The Emerging Role of Salaried Physicians: An Organizational Proposal." *The Journal of Public Health Policy* (September 1982): 284-292.

This article is a plea to begin a national association of salaried physicians. The authors maintain that at least 50% of all physicians in 1980 received at least partial payment in the form of a salary. Kahn and Orris say this new association would offer a well-needed alternative to "The AMA and its local groupings, traditional voices of medicine . . . historically locked into representing the AMA anachronistic cottage-industry physician." The authors claim such a new association is needed to promote working conditions, promotion and education of salaried doctors, as well as to define the interests of their patients and to improve nationwide health care. Lastly, the authors call for "eventual elimination of fee-for-service medical practice and institutions."

184. Kelly, Robert T. "American Medicine in the 1980s." *Minnesota Medicine* (April 1981): 207-209.

This article reflects AMA's concerns and interests at the beginning of the Reagan Administration. There is association optimism that Reagan will limit federal government interference with health care and rely more on the private sector for answers. The author, as a member of AMA's Board of Trustees, says AMA should take advantage of this opportune time and seek to defederalize and localize the health planning and PSRO programs. Dr. Kelly says the AMA realizes business and industry are up-in-arms about the increasing cost of employee health benefits and seek voluntary efforts, together with business and industry, to plan and implement joint cost-restraint approaches.

185. Kogan, Richard J. "Life, Death and Money - The Pharmaceutical Industry." *Vital Speeches* LVI(20) (August 1, 1990): 628-630.

The author, as Chairman of the Pharmaceutical Manufacturers Association, provides a defense of the pharmaceutical industry in this address to his association. Mr. Kogan cites the many contributions which drugs have made in health care. He covers the use of antibiotics and vaccines in eliminating infectious diseases and the costs saved in productivity alone. Mr. Kogan points out that drugs shorten hospital confinement, eliminate the needs for some surgery and make many new forms of advanced surgery more successful. The author accounts for the extensive R & D being conducted and for any new drugs under testing now for Alzheimer's, Parkinson's, osteoporosis, osteoarthritis, hypertension, arrhythmia, congestive heart failure and other illnesses. Mr. Kogan points out the risky investment, total costs and many years to develop a new drug. He claims that drugs actually cost less than in 1967, after adjustments for inflation. The author defends against government and third-party insurers who target the pharmaceutical industry for cost containment. Mr. Kogan concludes with the statement that the drug industry must be allowed to make money to cover risks and that the industry should be considered part of the solution to America's health care costs.

186. Loop, Floyd P. "Modern Medicine, An Index of American Civilization." *Vital Speeches* LVIII (9) (February 15, 1991): 269-272.

Dr. Loop, Chairman of the Board of Governors and CEO of The Cleveland Clinic, delivered this address to the City Club Forum in Cleveland, Ohio on November 30, 1990. The author provides his view of modern medicine -- why it's so expensive, who pays for it and what we can do to make it more equitable, efficient and less costly. The article provides excellent statistics on costs, payments, insurance coverage, health care and more. Dr. Loop specifically covers six major problems: 1) 32 million uninsured people; 2) drug abuse, poverty and teenage pregnancy; 3) the elderly, longer life and their higher health care costs; 4) financing health care and its administrative costs; 5) excess number of specialists versus primary care physicians; and 6) quality and effectiveness of some treatments. The author concludes with the corrective intentions of Health and Human Services, as well as his own prescription for action by Congress, business, individuals, and government. Dr. Loop warns that nationalizing health care will not stop rising costs nor diminish public expectations. He states that America has a culture which values the individual and personal rights and that our health care reflects that culture. "Our problems occur in trying to reconcile the value of medical advances in the context of social change."

187. Lundberg, George D. "The New American Medical Association, A Rededication to Excellence." *Journal of the American Medical Association* 236(8) (August 22/29, 1986): 1038-1040.

This article, taken from the proceedings of the June 1986 AMA annual convention, summarizes the association's new initiatives undertaken with a rededication to excellence in providing the best possible patient care. Dr. Lundberg says today's AMA will again focus on the centrality of science and education, along with long-standing involvement in clinical practice, politics, and economics as these affect physicians. The author provides examples of recent AMA actions to advance ethics, fight AIDS and tobacco, foster quality assurance and loyally defend members' professional rights. Lundberg concludes with AMA's initiatives to improve management, structure and strategic planning.

188. Mechanic, David. "Sources of Countervailing Power in Medicine." *Journal of Health, Politics, Policy and Law* 16(3) (1991): 485-499.

While the author does not address the AMA directly, he does discuss organized medicine's response to the increasing "corporatization" of medical practice. Mechanic reviews the assertions that there is a "loss of physician autonomy" and a "deprofessionalization and proletarianization of doctors" (p. 485) in this movement. However, he concludes that there is no significant change in the basic medical paradigm. "For-profit medicine has introduced constraints, but has not fundamentally changed the way doctors work" (p. 496), he asserts. In fact, Mechanic observes from the sociocultural perspective, "medicine is more central to the economy and more powerful than ever before" (p. 485).

189. Merz, Beverly. "American Medical Association: Speak Out About Need for Research on Animals." *American Medical News* (July 6/13, 1990): 9.

This very brief article addresses an issue which well represents the myriad topics the AMA must take action on in the interests of medical science. Specifically, the AMA has had to be an active proponent of the use of animals to support medical research. Support for this issue goes back to 1874. Today, advocacy involves countering aggressive animal rights activists and legal actions.

190. Minow, Newton N. "Report on Litigation to the American Medical Association House of Delegates." *Journal of the Tennessee Medical Association* 72(1) (January 1979): 46-52.

The author, as legal counsel for the AMA, delivered the message in this article to the AMA Interim Meeting of December 1978 in Chicago. Minow calls for unified action by organized medicine to counter the growing governmental intervention which threatens the freedom to practice medicine. The author, for example, cites AMA legal response to several Federal Trade Commission (FTC) actions and three suites by chiropractic associations against AMA. The article is highly useful in gaining an appreciation of AMA's perspective when defending against anti-trust measures that threaten association interests. In this article, the AMA charges the FTC with interfering with the profession's rights to set its own standards of ethical practices and to accredit medical schools. Specifically, the FTC ruled that AMA restrictions on physician advertising and its role in medical school accreditation both led to restraints on trade and violations of the 1890 Sherman Antitrust Act. In responding to chiropractic suits, the AMA had to defend against further charges of antitrust violation by precluding members from jointly practicing with unscientific cults. In this regard, the AMA classified its ethics guidelines in 1979 by announcing that any physician, on an individual judgment basis, may accept patient referrals from chiropractors.

191. Navarro, Vincente. "An analysis of the American Medical Association's recommendations for change in the medical care sector in the United States." *International Journal of Health Services.* 21(4) (1991): 685-696.

Professor Navarro charges the American medical care system is in a "profound crisis". In making this claim he provides numerous examples and supporting statistics. Furthermore, he charges the AMA with the duty to take a leadership role in resolving these challenges. Unfortunately, according to Navarro the recommendations offered by the AMA "bode ill for all patients and future patients, i.e., all citizens of the United States" (p. 686). He feels, "the AMA diagnosis of what ails our medical care system is wrong" (p. 689). America does not need more of the medicine as business mentality that has become so prevalent, but instead a return to medicine as a "call to serve" (p. 694). Navarro asserts that the AMA is no longer highly regarded by the American people nor by most practicing physicians. He sees instead the emergence of the role and leadership of the American College of Physicians who advocate a national health program.

192. Nelson, Alan. "American Medical Association Will Thrive as Our Umbrella Organization - If We Work At It." *American Medical News* (July 6/13, 1990): 7.

The author, as AMA President, addressed the association's House of Delegates with these thoughts on the organization's future. The AMA should strive to serve as an umbrella organization or a "convener" that brings diverse groups to take common action and use its political muscle. Dr. Nelson says the AMA must be known for promoting health for the public and not as an association representing medicine as a business. Nelson claims the AMA is more responsible and efficient and cites proactive accomplishments like its plan, Health Access America, as examples.

193. Nesbitt, Tom E. "The American Medical Association's Leadership Role." *Maryland State Medical Journal* (November 1974): 59-63.

The author, as Speaker of AMA's House of Delegates, provides his assessment of the accomplishments of AMA and the challenges to the profession, during a low point for AMA membership and fiscal resources. Dr. Nesbitt references the growth of medical specialty societies as a contributing factor to fragmentation. He furthermore maintains that national, state and country level AMA/medical society groups are often preoccupied with immediate issues, at the expense of commonly endeavoring to solve greater problems that impact them all. Nesbitt calls for improving communications among these groups and paying more attention to the needs of individual physicians and socioeconomical issues. Secondly, the author charges AMA with a leadership gap, implying the overall association has not proactively led efforts to manage change in health care and therefore government took action to fill the void. Nesbitt cites Medicare in 1965 and the enactment of PSROs as examples. The author challenges AMA to "act as builders of our own programs for progress rather than opposers of someone else's proposals. Acting in strength and in unity we can get the socioeconomic job done."

194. Nesbitt, Tom E. "What Doctors Can Do To Cut Medical Bills." *U.S. News and World Report* (August 14, 1978): 36-37.

The author, as President of the AMA, answers questions regarding the association's efforts in the late 1970s to influence doctors to go slow in raising their fees. Dr. Nesbitt says doctors have an incentive to make reasonable charges because runaway increases will accelerate the foreseen government intervention. The AMA reminds us that physician fees account for only 20% of the total healthcare dollar and that inflation and increased demand for services are powerful factors influencing fee increases. The AMA asked doctors to cut back the rate of increase in fee by 1 percent a year until it reaches 7 percent (compared to 13.5% in 1974). Simultaneously, The American Hospital Association, Federating American Hospitals and AMA asked hospitals to reduce its rate of increase by 2 percent a year for the next two years (compared to 16% in 1977).

195. Nutter, Donald O., Charles M. Helms, Michael E. Whitcomb, and W. Donald Weston. "Restructuring Health Care in the United States - A Proposal for the 1990s." *Journal of the American Medical Association* 265(19) (May 15, 1991): 2516-2520.

In addition to providing lead for the broad group that developed a proposal to reform the U.S. health care system, "Health Access America," the AMA asked its Medical School Section to sponsor restructuring plans separately. The authors were contacted by the Medical School Section to produce that plan. This article summarized their recommendations. While many recommendations are similar to "Health Access America," the Medical School Section plan includes proposals that may conflict with the former.

196. Petty, Roy. "Political Gains, Grassroots Problems." *Medical World News* 21(12) (June 9, 1980): 39-41, 45-46, 50, 52, 54.

Roy Petty's article describes changes in AMA's focus, resources and challenges since 1965—the "height of AMA's glory." The author maintains that the association's focus evolved "from a scientific and professional group into a predominantly political one... and has lost badly needed support from within the profession." Petty discusses membership problems, political battles, the growth of specialty societies and the personal impact of Dr. James Sammons -- the Association's flamboyant, outspoken leader. The article includes details on AMA's role with physician continuing education and lobbying strength. Petty implies that the AMA's problems may be common to most national groups and result largely from social, economic and political forces well beyond AMA's control.

197. Pinkney, Deborah S. "American Medical Association Wants IG Kusserow Fired Over Physician Fraud Probes." American Medical News (October 5, 1990): 1, 29.

This article illustrates the conflict that may arise between organized medicine and the federal government's Health and Human Services (HHS). Pinkney describes AMA's call for the resignation of the HHS Inspector General (IG). According to the association, the IG has taken an adversarial approach and has not acted fairly and responsibly in fraud investigations of physicians receiving Medicare and Medicaid reimbursement. As Pinkney points out, not all parties agree with AMA. Congressman Fortney "Pete" Stark, for example, defends the HHS IG and says their inspector "should get a medal for saving taxpayer fortunes."

198. Primich, Frank J. "What American Medical Association Has Not Done for Me Lately." *Medical World News* 19 (18) (September 4, 1978): 111.

This very short article by a New Jersey OB/GYN is highly critical, charging that AMA no longer is effective in defending American doctors from the interference of government. While Primich commends AMA for its journals and scientific programs, he claims AMA is giving in to Washington's push for national health insurance and activities to limit physician fees. Primich maintains that organizations like the Association of American Physicians and Surgeons and the Congress of County Medical Societies better represent physician interests, have taken more effective legal actions and therefore are more deserving of his financial support.

199. Rockefeller IV, Senator John D. "A Call for Action - The Pepper Commission's Blueprint for Health Care Reform." *Journal of the American Medical Association* 265 (19) (May 15, 1991): 2507-2510.

The Medicare Catastrophic Coverage Act of 1988 created the 15 member U.S. Bipartisan Commission on Comprehensive Health Care, or the Pepper Commission. With 12 congressional members and the presidential appointees, this commission was charged with assessing problems with the U.S. health care system and recommending legislation to resolve problems. This article provides an excellent summary of the commission's work and major recommendations. Readers interested in AMA's Health Access America, and national health insurance in general, should read and compare these various approaches to a highly complex issue.

200. Rogers, Frank A. "The American Medical Association: Yesterday, Today and Tomorrow." *The Journal of the Louisiana State Medical Society* 133(9) (September 1981): 129-135.

Dr. Rogers' article proposes "recapturing and revamping the AMA" to again become a defender of private medicine against further government intervention. The author charges the AMA for collaborating with government and allied health groups like the

American Nursing Association. Rogers claims we are quickly approaching socialized medicine which brings unnecessarily high health care costs. He further bemoans the loss of the physician's lead role in the health care team to nurses, hospital administrators and others. The author claims the AMA's significant loss in membership and declining support of private practice are results of poor leadership and a basic shift by the AMA to one regularly supporting government intervention. Rogers furthermore faults the Joint Commission on Accreditation of Hospitals, the Food and Drug Administration, The Department of Health and Human Services and others.

201. Sammons, James H. "Future Directions in American Medical Association Programming." *Journal of the American Medical Association* 253(11) (March 15, 1985): 1538-1585.

Dr. Sammons, as executive Vice President of the AMA, provides a summary of seven major areas of "increased emphasis" which the association will pursue over the near term. The article capitalizes a June 1984 report by the Board of Trustees entitled, "Future Directions and Resource Needs of the AMA, 1985-1987." Sammon says these "activities represent only a small portion of the association's work on more than 300 separate projects." The author then details initiatives taken in each area to: 1) preserve the quality of health care for the American people; 2) Help physicians respond to a changing practice environment; 3) strengthen relationships within the medical community; 4) revitalize the AMA's membership growth; 5) enhance the AMA's health policy development process; 6) expand the collection, analysis and dissemination of information related to medical practice concerns; and 7) secure AMA future. A valuable sidebar at the conclusion of the article states the four major purposes of the AMA, as established by the House of Delegates in 1981 and 1984. These purposes are to: 1) represent the medical progression; 2) provide information related to medicine; 3) establish, maintain and implement standards of conduct/performance; and 4) participate in establishing, maintaining and implementing medical education standards.

202. Sammons, James H. "Organized Medicine's Challenges Today: The Good, The Bad, and The Ugly." *Journal of MAG* 76 (July 1987): 499-502.

As Executive Vice President of the AMA, Dr. Sammons provides his impressions of what's good and bad in health care-- the challenges to today's organized medicine. On the negative side, the author discusses skyrocketing liability insurance premiums and organized medicine's fight for tort reform. Next, Dr. Sammons addresses the government's bundling of physician Medicare reimbursements into DRG payments. Sammons sees continued government intervention that will drive many doctors out of the Medicare program, thereby limiting the choice of physician by elder patients. Next, the author summarizes challenges involving CHAMPUS and then those in medical education. Dr. Sammons is worried about the profession no longer receiving the best and brightest of students, as these other concerns scare potential doctors to the world of business. Finally, the author cites several items of good news. Dr. Sammons sees improved cooperation among the AMA and state and local medical societies. He praises AMA and many others for developing and advocating the Health Policy Agenda for the American people. Lastly, Dr. Sammons praises AMA's new initiative for improving adolescent health care, citing the tremendous challenge faced by this "almost forgotten segment of our population."

203. Samuel, Frank E., Jr. "Health Care in America, Changes and Challenges." *Vital Speeches* LIII(11) (March 15, 1987): 335-337.

Mr. Samuel, as President of the Health Industry Manufacturers Association, provides an excellent speech on radical changes in U.S. health care in the 1980's. These changes, Samuel says, resulted from four basic factors: 1) problems with the U.S. federal deficit led to Medicare reforms in 1983 which initiated the diagnostic related groups (DRG) system and ended blanket reimbursement of whatever costs were incurred; 2) employers were able to pass more costs for medical insurance on to employees; 3) a surplus of doctors began to appear due to increased federal funding since 1965 of medical education; and 4) advances in medical technology led to more ambulatory care in the hospital, as well as expanded home health care programs; this means less expenditures in hospitals and more at lower cost, decentralized sites. In total, these changes mean tremendous growth in "managed care" at the most cost-effective site of care, real competition among physicians, further desire for controlling costs, and a drop from 1980s 95% fee-for-service payment to 1990s 40%. This in turn, will cause marginal providers to leave the market and a gradual check on cost growth. The author says that, given the right circumstances, we have experienced these cost reductions while still providing the patient choice of programs and quality care.

204. Samuel, Frank E., Jr. "Let's Make the Self-Care Revolution Work, Self-Medication in America's Future." *Vital Speeches* LIV(13) (April 15, 1988): 398-400 .

The author, as President of the Health Industry Manufacturer's Association, addresses the revolution in self-care in the U.S. Mr. Samuel says most Americans live to take charge with proven do-it-yourself diagnostic devices. The author provides numerous examples of the growth in these devices and their successful usage to date. Mr. Samuel then draws our attention to the "real excitement" in possibilities for the future, to include kits for strep throats, urinary tract infections and therapeutic drug monitoring. The author then forewarns us that the FDA, many physicians and others will continue as "institutionally conservative forces" often slow to encourage and endorse new self-care products. Yet advances will continue and, as long as manufacturers are responsible, the public will be eager consumers of more self-care devices.

205. Schoellhorn, Robert A. "Medical Technology, The Unseen Crisis." *Vital Speeches* LIV(4) (December 1, 1987): 122-125.

The author, CEO of Abbott Laboratories, warns "that our system's responses to demands for cost controls are now on a collision course with the new medical technologies being developed in response to public demands for more and better health care." Schoellhorn cautions that manufacturers, providers and purchasers must work together now to continue backing R & D on new technology. For example, physicians should get more involved in technology selection, but also pay close attention to cost savings factors in that selection. On the other hand, manufacturers should perform better marketing, not just selling the latest "gee whiz gadgets" but explaining which products can do what for controlling costs. Finally, Schoellhorn calls on government to rid itself of "regulations that serve as barriers to technology development."

206. Schwartz, Harry. "Surgeons Need to Join American Medical Association in a United Front." *American Medical News* (July 20, 1990): 23-24.

This brief article provides an example of how organized medicine can fragment into competing elements, rather than working together for their common interests. Specifically, Schwartz reviews the current feud between the AMA and American College of Surgeons, to include the sources of conflict. The author concludes with a call for unity.

207. Sherman, Sandra L. and Mark J. Segal. "American Medical Association Policy in the Resource-Based Relative Value Scale (RBRVS) and Related Issues." *Journal of the American Medical Association* 261(16) (April 28, 1989): 2386-2388.

This article represents AMA's strong intention to remain a key player in policy-making regarding Medicare physician payments. The authors summarize the association's position as stated in Report AA of the AMA Board of Trustees which was adopted December 6, 1988 by the House of Delegates. The report "supports an indemnity payment schedule based on an appropriate relative value scale (RVS) as the basis for a new Medicare physician payment system that would preserve physicians' autonomy, while eliminating the complexity of the customary, prevailing and reasonable (CPR) system."

208. Somerville, Janice. "Illinois Society will Continue American Medical Association Unification." *American Medical News* (April 20, 1990): 62.

This very brief article provides an example of how state medical society can be at odds with AMA and challenge the national association to take action. In this case, the Illinois State Medical Society threatened to deunify membership from the AMA by not requiring state society members to join the national association. Illinois voiced discontent over policy issues, scandal involving top AMA leadership, loss of sight regarding its mission, its administrative structure, managerial process and failure to express physicians' problems in Washington, D.C.

209. Stacey, James. "How the American Medical Association Develops Policy." *Journal of the American Medical Association* 250(11) (September 16, 1983): 1426-1427.

This article summarizes the process by which the AMA's House of Delegates meets twice yearly and acts on the many issues affecting health care. Stacey's article begins with pre-meeting actions and works through the system until completion. The author claims "few organizations are as rigorously democratic."

210. Todd, James S. "The American Health-Care System, Strengthen It, Don't Scrap It." *Vital Speeches* LVI (9) (February 15, 1990): 276-279.

The author, as Senior Deputy Executive Vice President of the AMA, provided this address to the National Education Association in San Antonio, Texas on October 5, 1989. Dr. Todd calls for strengthening our current health-care system rather than scrapping it for nationalized medicine or other drastic measure. The author cites the problems experienced by more socialized nations such as Britain, Holland and Canada. He states, "There is no country in the world that is currently at peace with its health-care system. They all have problems with financing. And they all have problems with delivery." Dr. Todd then provides the AMA's prescription to include expanding health insurance to all employed Americans, reform Medicare and Medicaid and establish state risk pools to help insurance companies cover those in poverty. The author then covers four common myths in U.S. health care and concludes with statements in American preference for individualism, limited government interventions, immediate treatment, high technology, and a greater role by their employer. This article is a good representation of the AMA's official thinking on our health-care problems and how to tackle them.

211. Todd, James S., Steven V. Seeking, John A. Krichbaum, J. D. Krichbaum, and Lynn K. Harvey. "Health Access America - Strengthening the U.S. Health Care System." *Journal of the American Medical Association* 265(19) (May 15, 1991): 2503-2506.

In 1982, the AMA and 172 other organizations initiated the Health Policy Agenda for the American people. This initiative, after five years of work by over 150 principles, led to a detailed prescription for improving access to affordable, high-quality health care. Now known as Health Access America, this prescription includes six fundamental principles on which to base specific policy, and 16 key points calling for action. This article describes what's wrong with our system now and what Health Access America prescribes as a fix. An example principle states that "affordable coverage for appropriate health care should be available to all Americans, regardless of income." One suggested way to accomplish those principles is a major Medicaid reform. The AMA estimates the proposal would cost the federal government about $21 billion annually, while costs to state governments, employees and individuals are additive.

212. Todd, James S. "Medical Progress, Good or Bad, So What?" *Vital Speeches* LVI(18) (July 1, 1990): 557-559.

Dr. Todd, as Senior Deputy Executive Vice President of the AMA, delivered this address to the United Way and Academy of Medicare of Cleveland on January 24, 1989. The author begins with the statement, "Medical progress good or bad matters little if we are out of step with social responsibility." Dr. Todd says we most question the notion of unlimited progress in medicine and realize delayed death results in more chronic illnesses or totally unresponsive patients sustained by artificial means. He continues that Americans worship technology and expect medicine to do everything scientifically possible for everybody all the time. Dr. Todd says we must begin to demand only what "needs to be done with reasonable expectation of benefits." We need to base medical decisions on moral considerations rather than just economic. For example, question spending a third of Medicare dollars on patients in the last year of life; or whether to spend billions on multiple transplants rather than for basic health-care needs. Dr. Todd challenges the public with four responsibilities: 1) know and practice good health habits; 2) do not make excessive demands on health-care systems, while being covered by insurance mechanisms that relieve individual responsibilities; 3) support legislation that provides entitlement to those who cannot do for themselves; and 4) start caring about the less fortunate.

213. Veatch, Robert M. "Professional Ethics: New Principles for Physicians?" *Hastings Center Report* 10(3) (June 1980): 16-19.

The author, Professor of medical ethics at the Kennedy Institute of Ethics, addresses AMA's 1980 draft revision of its medical ethics. Veatch provides us historical background, the AMA motives for revising their ethics and then reviews the new version, stating pros and cons in his opinion. The author says the previous version (1957) had measures affecting advertising and relating with chiropractic which led to lawsuits and the Federal Trade Commission's charge of restraint of trade. In addition, a revision was required to reflect that the physician is no longer the sole guardian of public health, that the principle of confidentiality should be strengthened, and that the physician must recognize his responsibilities which are linked to patient rights. The revised ethics, additionally binds the physician to deal honestly with patients and report unscrupulous colleagues. Moreover, the revision commits the physician to respect the law and ensures both patient and physician with freedom of choice. Veatch concludes with problem areas he sees as remaining with the revision and the author recommends further changes while praising AMA for these significant improvements.

214. Wagner, Lynn. "Hospitals Reject American Medical Association's Overture to Join Forces Over Medicare." *Modern Health Care* 20(7) (February 19, 1990): 6.

This very brief article illustrates the challenge sometimes faced by the AMA in finding allies to defend against government regulation of health care. Wagner refers to the AMA's January 1990 proposed alliance with the American Hospital Association and others to lobby against Medicare cuts. In this case, the hospital associations declined to join in coalition with AMA because labor groups and beneficiaries like the AARP felt the AMA does not support far-reaching reform of our health-care system that they and some Congressmen are seeking. Specifically, the AARP said that "linking publicly with the AMA would not advance its agenda of comprehensive health-care reform."

215. Wagner, Lynn. "Sullivan Denounces American Medical Association Ad Campaign." *Modern Health Care* 19(26) (June 30, 1989): 5.

This brief article illustrates the battles which are often fought between organized medicine and the U.S. Department of Health and Human Services. In this example, Secretary Louis W. Sullivan accuses the AMA of spreading false information in its campaign to discredit physician payment reform for Medicare, using expenditure targets. In its campaign, the AMA told the public that government targets would lead to the rationing of care and reduction of services.

216. Whelan, Elizabeth M. "Health Hoax and a Health Scare: Why Americans Don't Know the Difference." *Vital Speeches* LIV(2) (November 1, 1987): 57-61.

The speaker, as an Executive Director of The American Council on Science and Health, addresses how our public health priorities are confused. Whelan cites many examples to show that our government regulatory programs are misallocating the great majority of dollars and publicity towards controlling chemicals, food additives and other products which present minimal risks compared to the major causes of premature death. This, in turn, had led the public to be overly concerned about the strong health threats and under concerned as to preventive health which could be advanced through more emphasis on less risky life styles. Consequently, we assume natural is good and synthetic is evil. We prohibit needed insecticides and lose valuable crops. We virtually close down our nuclear energy programs although Three Mile Island's radiation to nearby residents equaled four puffs of a cigarette. We spend twice as much money through EPA for overkill on hazardous waste programs than for the National Cancer Institute to fight the leading cause of deaths. Or we fail to approve life saving drugs because the formula may carry intrinsic but small risks. Whelan calls on scientists, the media and general population to demand a more sensible approach to governmental regulating and health care priorities.

8

AMERICAN MEDICAL ASSOCIATION: MOVEMENT TOWARD THE FUTURE

The U.S. health care system is undergoing revolutionary changes induced by technological advances, financial pressures, changing public needs and desires, and growing ethical complexities. It is clear that this transformation will also change the place that physicians, and the American Medical Association, will occupy within the health care system of the future. Readings covered here deal with change and the future. Some look at AMA's perceptions and attitudes with respect to changes in the science and art of medicine. Others focus on AMA suggestions for improving hospitals and other health care institutions. Yet others concentrate on the future role of the AMA itself.

As the readings make clear, the Association, like any other entity, faces the perennial challenge of change: how to adapt with the times while keeping the best of the past. Articles point out the need for AMA activism in support of such causes as the fight against AIDS, adequate care for the elderly, improved trauma care, and higher quality health care. The role of the JCAHO (which the AMA belongs to) is given particular attention.

A number of articles call for a more flexible and efficient AMA, with active efforts at cost control, performance evaluation, strategic planning and management improvement. As one author points out, the basic challenge may be to get inherently individualistic physician professionals to take their organizational responsibilities seriously. According to these spokespersons, the Association must become more proactive in response to evolving national problems and sentiments.

Most of the authors feel that there is a future for the AMA - that the organization will continue to have a useful role to play within the nation's health care system. At the same time, there is a growing realization that past policies and behavior patterns will not suffice to keep the AMA viable. In a general but very real sense, the ultimate fate of the AMA - like that of the U.S. health care system itself - is in the hands of changing public needs and attitudes. If the AMA is to continue as an influential health care organization, it will have to transform itself as radically as the rest of the nation's medical care system in response to these changes.

(A) Books

217. Braverman, Jordon. *Crisis in Health Care.* Washington, DC: Acropolis Books, Ltd., 1978.

Published in 1978--the eve of the competitive and cost containment efforts begun in the Eighties--this work attempts to explain to the lay reader why a crisis in American health care exists, and what might be done to resolve it. The author is the former Director of Policy Analysis of the Health Policy Center at Georgetown University, and has previously worked with the Pharmaceutical Manufacturers Association, Blue Cross, and the American Pharmaceutical Association. For both intellectual and personal reasons (his brother being a physician), Mr. Braverman is particularly concerned with the likely transformation of the physician profession in the years to come.

The book is organized into nine chapters (totaling about 270 pages of text), and includes detailed references and a glossary of health care terminology. The chapters cover such topics as professional standards review organizations, health maintenance organizations, health care planning, medical malpractice insurance, private health insurance, and national health insurance.

In "The American Physician: A Tarnished Halo" (Chapter 2), the author asserts that "the American doctor and his manner of practice are being attacked today as never before" (p. 33). The growing image of doctors as greedy and dishonest has been fostered by legal challenges against American Medical Association restraints against physician advertising (which were ultimately struck down by the U.S. Supreme Court), and Federal Trade Commission investigations of alleged physician control of Blue Shield medical plans. Mr. Braverman concludes that "although the AMA's Principles of Medical Ethics say a physician should expose, without hesitation, illegal or unethical conduct by his colleagues, the good physicians have failed to police the bad ones" (p. 58).

The AMA is also portrayed as a chief obstacle to the systematic and independent oversight and management of physician practices. The Professional Standards Review Organizations (PSROs) that spread throughout the U.S. in the Seventies were initially opposed with great vigor by the AMA. So were HMOs. Throughout the Seventies, the AMA was found "opposing those health planning regulations which already have been published and which may be published in the future" (p. 135).

Even the national health insurance proposals supported by the AMA appear to be calculated to provide physicians with the greatest benefits and least controls. "Physicians fear any future national health insurance plan will assume the characteristics which critics attribute to the British National Health Service" (p. 230). The primary features of the AMA insurance plan include required private health insurance offerings to employees and subsidized private insurance for low-income and unemployed individuals.

In the long run, however, Mr. Braverman predicts that public opinion and financial pressures will reduce the political influence of the AMA and physicians, and transform the behavior of doctors with greater regulation and oversight.

218. Cray, Ed. *In Failing Health.* New York, NY: The Bobbs-Merrill Co., Inc., 1970.

Subtitled "The Medical Crisis and the AMA", this book is a critical account of the behavior of the American Medical Association in the health care sector. In thirteen chapters covering almost 250 pages, Ed Cray forcefully argues that the AMA is wedded to a medical status quo that condemns many of the poor and uninsured to misery. In its efforts to preserve a private sector-oriented, physician-dominated health care system (which is in fact inferior to health care systems in countries such as those of Western Europe), the AMA places the economic well-being of its members above the public good.

In the first three chapters, the author sets forth a vision of a fragmented, ineffective health care system that neglects the poor and reinforces persistent racism in the U.S. Health services providers are uncoordinated, underfunded and overburdened. People in need of health care are insufficiently organized for political action. In contrast, the AMA is a political juggernaut, capable of stopping any legislative or executive proposals it opposes through the carrots and sticks of its lobbying and campaign contribution programs. In Chapters IV and V ("Toxins and Antitoxins" and "A Hundred Thousand Evangelists"), Cray outlines what he feels is the generally reactionary political history of the AMA. The following chapter recounts the futile effort by the AMA to derail Medicare and Medicaid legislation (though, ironically, many of its members would find the programs to be financial bonanzas).

In "The Organized Crisis", the author provides evidence documenting his contention that since 1932 the AMA has intentionally created a national physician shortage (particularly with respect to general practitioners). Ensuing chapters detail the callousness of AMA-dominated physicians to the needs of the poor and minorities ("Cash and Carry Medicine"), the practices of patient-dumping and unnecessary surgery by profit-hungry doctors and hospitals ("One Drop at a Time"), and the promising but troubled neighborhood health centers sponsored by the Office of Economic Opportunity ("The Bronx Experiment").

In Chapters XI through XIII, Cray summarizes and generalizes his indictment of the AMA-dominated health care system. In particular, he criticizes what he sees as AMA opposition to group practice and other arrangements which would provide comprehensive care: "Under the guise of 'medical ethics', the profession has waged a long and still continuing battle to preserve traditional market practices which heavily favor the doctors' pockets" (p. 201).

The author concludes with a call for a national health insurance program which would provide comprehensive care for all citizens, praises the efforts in support of such legislation by such organizations as the United Auto Workers, and lists the most recent efforts by the AMA to defeat or coopt all such proposals. He also provides a blow-by-blow account of the successful AMA derailing of the nomination of John Knowles to be the Nixon Administration's Secretary of Health, Education and Welfare, as well as the eventual appointment of the almost-as-objectionable (to the AMA) Roger O. Egeberg. Despite the opposition, Cray declares that national health insurance is both inevitable and necessary if American medicine is to fulfill "within its capabilities the promise of life" (p. 245).

219. Duff, Raymond S. and August B. Hollingshead. *Sickness and Society*. New York: Harper and Row, 1968.

This book focuses on the relationship between the care of hospitalized patients and the social environment of a university and community hospital. While interesting to read and valuable in gaining insight into the ups and downs of hospital based medical practice, there is no specific discussion of the AMA in the book. However, if the reader is interested in organized medicine at the micro, i.e. institutional level during the 1960's heyday of medical practice, this is a book that should be read.

220. Ginzberg, Eli. *The Medical Triangle.* Cambridge, MA: Harvard University Press, 1990.

In this recently issued collection of previously published articles, Eli Ginzberg, an eminent scholar of health policy and Professor at Columbia University, further elaborates upon his often troubled and troubling vision of U.S. health care as it approaches the 21st Century. The twenty essays (covering almost three hundred pages) are divided into five sections: "The Changing Health System" (an overview of Dr. Ginzberg's concerns, particularly concerning medical profit-making and privatization); "Important Subsystems" (academic health centers, foundations, community health centers, and health care in New York City); "Medical Education, the Physician Supply and Nursing" (covering the named topics); "Patients' Needs and Resources" (including care for the poor, elderly and cancer patients); and "Health Agenda Issues" (cost containment and quality assurance challenges).

In "The Politics of Physician Supply", Dr. Ginzberg most directly addresses the present and possible future roles for physicians in American health care. The author begins with an account of the American Medical Association's historical efforts at professional reform that led to the Flexner Report and the heightened regulation (and numerical reduction) of medical schools. He points out that the AMA continued to advocate the restriction of physician supply well into the Sixties, until the Federal Government adopted legislation promoted by Senator Lister Hill (D - Alabama) to subsidize medical education in 1963.

From 1963 to 1971, the national government made further efforts to expand the supply of physicians, with such measures as the establishment of the National Health Service Corps (1970), the Health Professions Educational Assistance Act (1971), and the Area Health Education Centers program (1971). By 1968 (with a prominent article in the Journal of the American Medical Association by F. J. L. Blasingame, Executive Vice President), the AMA was already beginning to revise its position to one of supporting increased medical school enrollment. Ironically enough, however, opinion by the mid-Seventies was already beginning to shift again, to the position that the emerging problem would be one of a physician surplus rather than shortage. The GEMENAC Report, released in 1980 (and attacked by the AMA for alleged methodological shortcomings), advocated sharp cutbacks in medical school admissions. The AMA was not willing to concur with this new orientation until 1986.

Dr. Ginzberg concludes that "the politics of the physician supply has revealed that the parties of primary interest have been the members of the medical profession and the medical education fraternity. Further, it has revealed the influence of pseudo-science, inasmuch as most studies of the demand for and supply of physician personnel have proved to be egregiously wrong, often within as short a time as five years" (p. 195). Ultimately, the proper physician supply must be determined by broadly political decision making, not statistical models.

221. Jones, Rochelle. *The Supermeds.* New York, NY: Charles Scribner's Sons, 1988.

The central topic in this work is the corporatization of American medicine. The book's subtitle, "How the Big Business of Medicine is Endangering Our Health Care", accurately indicates Ms. Jones' critical attitude toward the changes in health care in the latter Seventies and Eighties. In nine chapters and approximately 225 pages, the author outlines the problem ("Good- bye to Dr. Marcus Welby", "Getting Less but Paying More Too", "The No-Care Zone", and "The Lovely Gleam of Gray Gold") and concludes with suggestions on "Taming the Corporation".

By and large, Ms. Jones is sympathetic to the American Medical Association, portraying the organization as a force for traditional, patient-centered medicine that is slowly losing the fight against profit-hungry corporations (the "supermeds") that will erode the doctor-patient relationship in pursuit of the dollar sign (or the dollar savings). But AMA surveys show that younger physicians are themselves more likely to support the supermeds.

At a 1986 AMA conference on "the revolution in the health care industry", the Association belatedly recognized the threat that the supermeds were posing. "For the past twenty years AMA leaders had been warning doctors that their biggest threat came from the federal government and its support of 'socialized medicine' through the funding of health care programs for the poor and elderly. As the AMA fought the federal government, however, they failed to perceive that the emerging health care conglomerates posed a far larger danger to the medical profession" (p. 69). In the author's estimate, "the private practitioners who make up the bulk of the American Medical Association membership are becoming an anachronism" (p. 71).

If nothing is done, the future of American medicine will be bleak. AMA surveys show that doctors' incomes are already stagnating, and future physicians are more likely to be forced to adopt marketing and business techniques (that neglect the true interests of the patient) in order to survive. The AMA also points out that in 1985, 25.7% of doctors were employed by prepaid health plans, while another 20% were salaried hospital practitioners. Prospective payment systems are also being used by hospitals and payers to change physician practice styles and ration care. Given all of this, it is not surprising that other AMA research reveals that "medical school applications are falling because of fear that the financial rewards of becoming a physician are dwindling" (p. 210).

222. Knowles, John, H. *Hospitals, Doctors, and the Public Interest.* Cambridge, MA: Harvard University Press, 1966.

As the General Director of the Massachusetts General Hospital, Mr. Knowles edits a collection of lectures sponsored by the Lowell Institute and presented at MGH in 1963. The emphasis of these lectures was on "The Hospital's Responsibility to the Community." In discussing the role of the hospital as a social influence over socioeconomic issues of medical care, education, and the future of health care in the community, this book was written for the layman and the medical professional alike.

There were a few of the lectures that mentioned the AMA, but those that did discussed the historical positions more than the AMA's present ones. E.D. Churchill, M.D. mentions that "the prime reason for the organization of the AMA in 1847 was to elevate the standard of medical education" (Medical Education in the Hospital, p. 224). Others included the role of the curriculum to interns and residents. J. Pollack, M.D. compliments the AMA for its "valuable contribution (The Voice of the Consumer, p. 181) to the rights of organizing independent practices and their payment plans."

223. Mechanic, David. *From Advocacy to Allocation.* New York, NY: The Free Press, 1986.

Subtitled "the evolving American health care system," this book is a collection of articles dealing with the ongoing changes in U.S. health services delivery. The author has published frequently on health policy and sociology in the last twenty years. The relatively brief (about 230 pages) book is divided into four parts: issues in health policy; the promotion of health, illness behavior, and the management of illness; the health professions; and the health of special populations.

In "Changing Conceptions of the Physician and Public Conceptions of Medicine" (Chapter 7), the author states that more and more Americans have negative images of doctors, and disunity and conflict are steadily growing within the ranks of physicians, causing problems for the American Medical Association. "Existing trends suggest that fragmentation among doctors will increase and perhaps lead to greater acrimony within the profession. . . . The American Medical Association has increasing difficulty in formulating policies that hold its membership together" (p. 136).

224. Smith, D. B. and Arnold D. Kaluzny. *The White Labyrinth*, Second Edition. Ann Arbor, MI: Health Administration Press, 1986.

This book is subtitled "A Guide to the Health Care System". It represents an effort by two eminent scholars of health care administration to provide a conceptual framework for understanding the structure and processes of the U.S. health care system. As such, the book does not attempt to provide the reader with a full understanding of recent health services research, or practical guidelines for management. It is, in the fullest sense, a work of organizational theory.

For all of that, The White Labyrinth is remarkably concise and tightly organized. Only slightly over two hundred pages in length, the book is divided into three parts, each with three chapters, and a fairly detailed references section at the end. Part I ("Creating the Labyrinth") describes how the U.S. health care system was developed, and the result of its particular characteristics. "Working Within the Labyrinth", the second part, moves the focus from the system as a whole to the organizational and individual level. Part III, "Escaping the Labyrinth", provides a general discussion of possible ways in which the health care system might be improved through change.

Smith and Kaluzny suggest that the American Medical Association has been, for better and for worse, a force for establishing a unitary and homogeneous medical profession--a key element of "the white labyrinth". Beginning with the AMA's foundation in 1847, the Association and its adherents engaged in a crusade "to control medical education and restrict the practice of medicine to persons who practiced as they did" (p. 20). The AMA also supported the Carnegie Foundation's study by Abraham Flexner that called for a more standardized, scientific American medical education and practice. As a result, now "a single, homogeneous profession exercises a virtual monopoly over the provision of services" (p. 21).

The very success of the AMA and the physician profession, however, have begun to generate counter forces. The control by a physician elite over health care is now being increasingly challenged by hospitals, the government, and other health care professionals, including those in nursing and allied health. The large, specialized and centralized "labyrinth" that the AMA and physicians did so much to create must now be transformed into a more decentralized and participatory health care system that is oriented toward community and patient interests.

225. Turner, Bryan S. *Medical Power and Social Knowledge.* London: Sage, 1987.

This insightful medical sociology text concerns itself with the identity of medicine as a sociological phenomenon. In particular the book explores the relationship between knowledge and power in the social distribution of health and illness. Additionally the role of medical discourse as the foundation of medical power is examined. Specific treatment of the AMA is quite sparse for a book on this topic, in fact, the AMA is only mentioned twice. However, in one of these passages the author does assert, "The AMA has been successful in preventing the development of a centralized, public system of health-care delivery." He cites several examples of how the AMA has worked closely with the insurance industry to "oppose all moves to introduce a compulsory national insurance scheme" (p.190).

(B) Articles

226. Affeldt, John E. "The JCAH and Voluntary Accreditation." *Journal of Oral Surgery* 39 (1981): 94-96.

Dr. Affeldt, as President of the JCAHO, describes the hospital accreditation structure and voluntary process as a highly successful alternative to government regulation. The article traces the Commissioner's history and accomplishments, as well as how accreditation standards are developed or revised.

227. "AMA, The Future of Medicine, A Scenario Analysis." *Journal of the American Medical Association* (July 3, 1987): 258.

AMA's Council on Long Range Planning and Development shares its forecast for U.S. Medicine through the year 2000 and what AMA must do to remain successful in the changing environment. The Council's methodology uses three different scenarios, with widely differing assumptions on the health of the U.S. economy. Based on those scenarios, analysis is performed and implications for AMA are developed. This is followed by possible AMA responses to ensure its success into the next millennium.

The AMA forecasts a definite continuing need for its association. It sees a need to be more successful in earning income through various enterprises that would permit delimiting increases in membership dues. The AMA finds it essential to work with other associations of organized medicine to reduce duplication of effort and each, for economy, better focus its efforts on fewer, top priority activities. The AMA furthermore encourages mergers of closely related medical societies.

The AMA also sees the need to increase its visibility as a more responsive, proactive leader in health policy through better communication with physicians, the media, and the general public. The Council, furthermore, prescribes enforcing professional standards for AMA membership, continuing to recruit medical students, residents, and young physicians as new members, and strengthening its planning process.

Finally, the Association calls for adopting a more flexible structure with all AMA sections evaluated for performance. Significant cost reductions must be sought. In summary, the AMA sees a future where competition among physicians and among medical societies increases and where income constraints necessitate well planned, better focused and efficient attention to priority activities. "The AMA must change itself to succeed in the future."

228. "AMA's Role in the Fight Against AIDS." *American Medical News* (May 11, 1990): 19.

This brief editorial is a good summary of the Association's extensive efforts to support the nation's war against AIDS. The author includes AMA's support of legislators, public information programs, and issuance of extensive policy reports containing hundreds of recommendations, including the call for a broad national policy to fight AIDS.

229. Bell, Clark W. "JCAHO Missed Opportunity." *Modern Health Care* (October 28, 1988): 31.

The author chides the JCAHO for not responding in writing to the October 12, 1988 article in the *Wall Street Journal* which criticized the JCAHO. Bell reminds us the JCAHO is powerful, in that failure to accredit a hospital can bankrupt the institution which then cannot receive the Medicare reimbursements. While the JCAHO rarely denies accreditation and rarely conducts surprise inspections, says Bell, it is one of the most powerful groups in healthcare and has made many progressive changes in upgrading standards at hospitals, HMOs, nursing homes, hospices, outpatient clinics and other alternative care settings.

230. Berger, Sally and Susan K. Sudman. "Making Total Quality Management (TQM) Work." *Healthcare Executive* (March/April 1991): 22-25.

This article challenges hospital CEOs to make TQM work. The authors cite several cases in hospitals where quality programs floundered. They then provide five warning signals to help CEOs to recognize problems in their TQM programs. The authors caution CEOs to marry the TQMs "change strategy" to overall management strategies and measure results in terms of care, service and costs. The TQM definition should not be too narrowly defined, but rather include clinical outcome, service to the customer and management structure and process. TQM must seek interdepartmental interpretation and involve all departments and levels of an organization. Finally, the authors suggest to CEOs that an effective TQM program may take longer to implement than the average tenure of today's CEO.

231. Breo, Dennis L. "Dr. Todd Looks Toward AMA's Future." *Journal of the American Medical Association* 265 (4) (June 26, 1991): 3306-3307.

Breo addresses several key initiatives and concerns of Dr. Todd, AMA's Executive Vice President. The author says Dr. Todd seeks to better focus AMA on doing fewer things better. The Association must help the nation define the basic level of health care that it wants to provide all citizens; such an AMA initiative exists in the comprehensive Health Access America Program, advocated in 1991. The AMA seeks to be highly influential in matters such as medical costs, quality care, education, ethics, science, public health, and manpower. Todd challenges doctors as "marvelous individualists" to close ranks and take effective collective action to help physicians practice quality medicine and retain their ability to care for patients.

232. Breo, Dennis L. "Dr. Todd, Newly Named EVP, Will Work for Friendlier, Wiser AMA." *Journal of the American Medical Association* 264 (July 25, 1990): 514-516.

The author provides insights on the Association's new chief based on an interview with Dr. Todd. The new Executive Vice President states, "At AMA, all our activities -- from accreditation to legislation to publications -- are intended to create an environment in which the physician can treat the patient as well as possible." Specifically, Dr. Todd's agenda for AMA includes: 1) making AMA a friend of those it serves -- physicians, patients, and government; 2) better focusing AMA efforts and doing fewer things better; 3) registering AMA visibility as the champion of professionalism and with a more proactive and aggressive role in Washington; and 4) managing efficiently and improving non-dues revenues. Dr. Todd sees universal access to medical care as a given and is proud of AMA's "Health Access America" proposal.

On other topics, Dr. Todd regrets stand-alone tactics of specialty associations and calls for subjecting medical services to a benefit-user analysis, whereby we better allocate costly health care to those who will realize the most benefits. His top goal is to "preserve rational physician autonomy" by ensuring physicians are free to make medical decisions best for the patient.

233. Burda, David. "JCAHO to Review Managed Care." *Modern Healthcare* (March 11, 1988): 6.

This very brief article describes the growing role of the JCAHO in accrediting managed-care HMOs and PPOs under contract for state governments like Minnesota, Hawaii, Kansas, and Pennsylvania. While managed-care institutions become major providers of health care, federal regulations require state Medicaid programs that were managed-care plans to hire private reviewers.

234. Burda, David. "JCAHO Dismisses Article." *Modern Healthcare* (October 21, 1988): 9.

This short article covers the JCAHO response to an October 12, 1988 *Wall Street Journal* article by Mr. Walt Bogdanich -- a Pulitizer Prize winner for reporting on healthcare problems. Burda gives to JCAHO claims that the Wall Street article was "sensational journalism." The Bogdanich article claimed the JCAHO only refused the accredit 0.3% of 3,500 hospitals surveyed in 1986 and 1987.

Furthermore, says Bogdanich, the JCAHO is slow in reporting deficiencies to hospitals, accredits many with quality-of-care deficiencies, keeps survey details confidential from consumers and is hesitant to take actions against hospitals.

235. Burda, David. "JCAHO Survey Finds Concern Over Standards." *Modern Healthcare* (April 9, 1990): 54.

This very short article provides the results of an opinion poll of 923 hospital CEOs by the JCAHO. The poll showed CEOs were most concerned about JCAHO content and focus of accreditation standards. Others said standards were too general and open for interpretation. Still other CEOs said they were concerned that the public would misinterpret survey information leading to false conclusions about quality care. While the JCAHO uses such opinion polls to work on improving survey effectiveness and efficiency, 53% of CEOs said the JCAHO's overall performance during the past five years got worse or stayed the same.

236. Burda, David. "JCAHO Ending Managed-Care Accreditation." *Modern Healthcare* (May 28, 1990): 3.

This brief article describes the end to the JCAHO's two years of evaluating managed-care institutions. Of the 590 HMOs, the JCAHO had performed only 13 accreditations in this two year period. Reportedly, HMOs felt the commission's standards were too stringent and inflexible. Termination of this program leaves the JCAHO with five accreditation programs -- long-term care, general and psychiatric hospitals, other psychiatric facilities, ambulatory-care facilities and home-care organizations. For future accreditations of managed care facilities, National Committee for Quality Assurance now is the preeminent player.

237. Cooper, Theodore. "Foundations, Traditions and Directions in U.S. Health Care: Technology and Social Policy." *Vital Speeches* LVII (November 15, 1990): 79-81.

The speaker, as CEO of the Upjohn Company, addresses the "three driving forces" affecting U.S. health care -- costs, technology, and social expectations. Cooper states we are in a period when the cost-factor is predominant and there is too much emphasis on economics for solutions. Cooper claims technology is way ahead of our social policy in such areas as care of the elderly. The author speaks to the need for strong funding of biomedical research, the many spin-off advances now being realized and the need to attract our brightest young people to scientific research. He concludes with a general prescription for reform of U.S. health care.

238. Cooper, Theodore. "How High a Priority Will Society Accord to Health Care?" *Vital Speeches* LIII (February 1, 1987): 242-245.

The author, as Vice Chairman of the Board of Directors, the Upjohn Company, addresses the growth of U.S. health care, with public policy now driven by cost containment. Cooper points out that Americans behave very differently as a group compared to individuals' values regarding health care. While the group votes for HMOs and against expensive treatment for aged people with little remaining life expectancy; the individual American demands the best technology, their own specialist of choice, and no limitations on care.

The author believes our health care policy ought to have a realistic attitude about assuring quality, controlling the rate of growth in expenditures, developing a favorable mix of services, and creating more uniformity throughout the system. Cooper says Americans, however, want a two-tiered system; some people will give up freedom of choice for lower costs and enroll in HMO programs. Others will not. The author says growth in health care will continue because of factors such as the push to cover the underinsured and uninsured, the aging of Americans and the discovery and demand for new medical technologies and drugs.

239. Goldsmith, Martha F. "AMA House of Delegates Adopts Comprehensive Measures on AIDS." *Medical News and Perspectives* 258(4) (July 24/31, 1987): 425-426.

This article is an excellent example of AMA policy issued to assist association members, government and the public in seeking solutions to a serious health problem. Goldsmith's article summarizes AMA's June 1987 report, entitled "Prevention and Control of AIDS." The report makes 17 specific recommendations for action, as well as three resolutions adopted by the House of Delegates. Although brief, the article illustrates just how complex such policy can be and reflects the immense amount of effort the AMA is willing to take in helping to solve major illnesses.

240. Grimaldi, Paul L. "How New Physician Fee Schedule Will Work." *Healthcare Financial Management* (September, 1991) :58-75.

Dr. Grimaldi discusses the Healthcare Financing Administration's (HCFA) new Medicare fee schedule for physicians will break physician services into three components: physical work, practice expenses, and malpractice expenses. HCFA intends the new fee schedule to reduce and more equitably distribute Medicare expenditures for physician services. For healthcare organizations, the new fee schedule may mean changes in revenue collections, revisions to coding and billing systems, and greater competition between physicians and outpatient hospital services. The AMA has been critical of this program and has specifically chided the proposal that this plan will reduce overall Medicare physician payments by three billion dollars.

241. Hampton, Oscar P., Jr. "The Challenge of the Trauma Problem to Organized Medicine." *The Journal of Trauma* 10(11) (1970): 926-931.

Dr. Hampton's article calls on organized medicine, from national AMA level to local county medical societies, to aggressively support government and volunteer actions to reduce casualties to trauma. The author specifically requests immediate action to bring about adequate safety regulations, effective community level emergency medical services, enhanced continuing education for physicians in life-saving techniques, and supportive regional categorization of hospitals according to emergency medical capabilities.

242. Holthaus, David. "JCAHO Confidentiality Undergoes Public Scrutiny." *Hospitals* (April 20, 1989): 56-57.

This article provides an example of how Congress can impact the U.S. health care system by interceding in the voluntary, self-regulated quality control process driven by the Joint Commission on Accreditation of Health Care Organizations (JCAHO). In this case, the General Accounting Office, at the request of Representative Pete Stark from California, was tasked to investigate whether JCAHO surveys are ensuring quality health care. In the process, legislation may be passed which requires the JCAHO to disclose detailed survey information to the publicly-funded Health Care Financing Administration. The JCAHO, and its members such as the AMA, fear that survey information disclosed to the public will be misunderstood, and that physicians will be reluctant to discuss quality care during accreditation surveys, "out of fear of lawsuits or reprisals."

243. Kissick, William L. "Health Care in the '80s." *Vital Speeches* LII (7) (January 15, 1986): 213-218.

The author, as the Pepper Professor of Public Health and Preventive Medicine at the University of Pennsylvania, addresses major changes in health care in the '80s, consequences of those changes and critical choices each of us face. The major changes Professor Kissick reviews are those in personnel, facilities, R & D, financing and organization. The author talks about the six million plus workers in health care, the surplus of physicians and medical schools. He then looks at excess hospital bed capacity. Third, the post World War II advances in biomedical research and technological innovations are covered. Fourth, Kissick accounts for changes in health insurance and financing of health care. Fifth, the author looks at corporate restructuring of health care organizations, HMOs, PPOs, hospital systems and urgent care centers. After reviewing these major changes, Mr. Kissick speaks to their consequences. The need to improve productivity; aspects of competition among medical schools and physicians; the continued coalescing of hospitals, physicians and insurance companies; the channeling of health care into profitable, market driven programs; and rise of salaried practitioners versus independent professionals. Professor Kissick concludes with five initiatives we all should take: change living habits and improve self-care; choose the right health care provider and insurance for your needs; choose the right treatment means and value as an involved consumer; join special interest groups that best represent your needs; and communicate with politicians to make known your needs and voting power.

244. Koska, Mary T. "New JCAHO Report Assesses Hospitals' Standards Compliance." *Hospitals* (January 5, 1991): 32-33.

This article concerns the new annual report by the JCAHO which summarizes the performance of over 5,000 hospitals in complying or not with accreditation standards. The first report, entitled "Hospital Accreditation Statistics 1986-1989", indicates that hospitals with the most severe resource problems also find it more difficult to comply with accreditation standards. The author quotes the JCAHO President, Dr. Dennis O'Leary, "...many hospitals seem to be on a collision course with standards. You have a steadily rising cascade of requirements at the same time that Medicare and private-sector payments are being curtailed." This new report not only allows hospitals to compare themselves with others but also will be used in business by such users as corporate health care purchasers. Koska's article includes a graphic which shows ratings of compliance by selected area, for example 4.9% of hospitals were rated as "non-compliance" in monitoring and evaluation of special care services.

245. Koska, Mary T. "JCAHO: Pilot Hospitals' Input Updates Agenda for Change." *Hospitals* (January 5, 1990): 50-52, 54.

This article describes the JCAHO's program for developing "clinical indicator sets" of data for specialties like anesthesia and obstetrics. Based on inputs from many participating hospitals, aggregate data are compiled, analyzed and returned to hospitals to help them measure how they are performing. This Agenda for Change initiative should eventually provide a significant analytical tool in facilitating quality assurance improvements.

246. Koska, Mary T. "JCAHO Gets Lukewarm Reviews from its CEO Opinion Survey." *Hospitals* (May 5, 1990): 46, 48-49.

Koska's article provides the results of a JCAHO survey sent to 923 hospital CEOs to obtain feedback on the accreditation program. The feedback presented an overall "lukewarm" rating by CEOs. Example criticism included charges that accreditation standards were too vague and inconsistently applied. CEOs felt better focus and content of standards needed the most improvement. Koska's article includes the top 15 areas of most concern to CEOs.

247. Martini, Carlos J. "The Long Shadow of Flexner: A Prolonged Polemic in Assessing Outcomes in Medical Education." *Journal of the American Medical Association* 262(8) (August 25, 1989): 1008-1010.

The author briefly reviews the history of the Flexner influence on the accreditation process and argues that the philosophical underpinnings which are grounded in process criteria could be missing the mark in the improvement of medical education. Dr. Martini offers an orientation toward outcomes measurement as more appropriate and more promising for a revitalization of medical education assessment.

248. Meyer, Harris. "American Medical Association, Rand, Academic Centers Near Practice Guidelines Accord." *American Medical News* (February 9, 1990): 1, 40.

The federal government is pushing for the development of practice parameters to help health care providers minimize delivery of unnecessary care. Meyer's article describes a joint effort by the AMA, the Rand Corporation and eight academic medical centers to develop "clinical guidelines" for procedures such as coronary artery bypass and cataract surgery.

249. Oglesby, D. Kirk, Jr. "The JCAHO: Straight Talk from an Insider." *Hospitals* (August 20, 1990): 26.

The author, as AHA commissioner to the JCAHO, comments on the responsiveness and future role of the accreditation committee. Oglesby acknowledges that much criticism has been made regarding the survey process, timeliness of reports and assistance to hospitals. The author claims the JCAHO is placing better trained people in the field and will listen closely to those surveyors on how to improve the process. Oglesby says a basic concern remains in determining the true value of the accreditation program. Other challenges include the demand to release more survey data to the public, to reduce paperwork requirements and red tape and to maintain a close relationship with federal and state governments. The author thinks the JCAHO should continue to play a major role in measuring quality performance in health care because of its history and abilities. This role "will require compromise, increased knowledge and some shift in emphasis."

250. O'Leary, Dennis S. "The Joint Commission's Agenda for Change." *Journal of Medicine* 76 (July of 1987): 503-507.

Dr. O'Leary, as President of the JCAHO, describes the new initiatives under the Commission's "Agenda for Change." The agenda includes these distinct programs: an effort to revamp the survey process to evaluate whether an organization "does" provide quality health care (versus capability); and initiative to improve communications and professional relationships between the JCAHO and providers, government and business; and an effort to expand the Commission's education and consultation services. This article keys in the first initiative, where the Commission hopes to use new "clinical indicators" and continuous on-line data and analyses to evaluate and assist with "desired ends" regarding patient care. If successful, a health care organization could readily compare its performance to external and internal expectations (norms) and know how it is performing in actually providing quality care, by comparison to data in other institutions.

251. Robinson, R. G. "JAMA at 100." *New Zealand Medical Journal* 96(738) (August 24, 1983): 654.

This very short article praises the centennial and accomplishments of JAMA. Robinson underlines the importance of JAMA in the very survival and growth of the AMA. Robinson comments on several of its first 13 editors and on the journal's tremendous revenue-making importance with the golden years of advertising revenues peaking in the 1960s. The author points out that "most medical associations have come to realize that the standing of their medical journal is something that must be maintained if the medical association is to exercise the leadership its constitution implies."

252. Scearse, Patricia. "Accreditation: The Good, The Bad and The Ugly." *Journal of Professional Nursing* 5(3) (May/June 1989): 123, 168.

This short article questions the validity and value of health care institution accreditation, given recent findings by federal and state inspectors. The author indicates the Health Care Financing Administration (HCFA) is now just catching up to its 1972 congressional mandate to monitor work of the JCAHO. In the process, findings show the JCAHO accredited 99.7% of 3,500 hospitals inspected in 1986 and 87, while as many as one-third of those hospitals accredited were found to have serious problems by state inspectors. Scearse questions whether the JCAHO is impartial and appropriate in accreditation decisions, given the fact that the principal source of revenue for the JCAHO is the members who hope to obtain accreditation. The author foresees hospitals and educational institutions, which receive federal funds, becoming the likely objects of increased scrutiny.

253. Winters, Robert C. "Picking Sides in Health Care's Quality Revolution." *Vital Speeches* LVIII (7) (January 15, 1991): 211-214.

The speaker, as CEO of the Prudential Insurance Company, addresses the meaning and pursuit of better quality in U.S. health care.

Winters says the demand for better quality must come from "outside" (government) as well as the "inside" (hospital quality teams). Government, for example, now maintains automated data files to identify problem doctors and other health practitioners. Winters calls on the government to fund more research in health care outcomes research, to help consumers (patients) make smarter decisions on doctor and treatment selection. Consumers are now waking up and demanding more devices and their right to call the shots. At the same time, insurance companies are developing managed care networks that influence prices and treatments. They are approving providers, negotiating reimbursements and screening hospitals. Their goal is to answer the quality and appropriateness of care. Winters concludes with three tenets for a new health care "quality manifesto." First, quality can be improved. Second, better quality can be less expensive. Third, our definition of quality can be more exact.

EPILOGUE:

Interview with Lester King, M.D.

Medical historian and former Senior Editor of
the Journal of the American Medical Association

AUTHORS: What is your overall historical perspective on the American Medical Association?

KING: Ostensibly, the AMA was started in 1847 to raise the level and quality of physician education. There were too many doctors and too many diploma mills; the profession was diluted. But in effect the Association became a straightforward union, to restrict entry and competition; it really wasn't a high-minded enterprise. President Davis (Nathan Smith Davis, a founder and historian of the AMA) always claimed that the organization was high-minded. But his claims were personally self-serving, and haven't born out by what actually happened.

A lot of what happened was due to other things. Technology changed over time. During the mid-1850s, there was no money for doctors in medicine. Things just got too expensive for the old proprietary system. So there was a tendency for medical schools to associate with universities for more revenue. That is really where the true impetus for medical education came from. The AMA supported university affiliates except it tended to produce two types of physicians—university affiliates and practitioners. It was a town and gown conflict. The AMA had ties to both camps. But eventually the AMA came down on the side of practicing rather than academic doctors. Between 1885 and 1910, elitism took great steps forward, and specialization began.

AUTHORS: To what extent does the AMA influence public policy on health care?

KING: That's not a simple question so you won't get a simple answer. the AMA is really schizophrenic with respect to power and politics. It has influence, yet, in principle, it opposes political influence over health politics. Certainly, the AMA has political power, but the organization doesn't have a temperament well suited for the political process.

263

AUTHORS: How has that affected the AMA's activities?

KING: Well, things may be changing rapidly now. I don't have real firsthand knowledge. But, I have a perception - I think if you go over history of the Journal, the quarrels over homeopathy are typical for AMA politics. Some doctors hated homeopathy because it took away business, and was not "scientific". The AMA's hand was forced when the homeopaths lobbied the Michigan legislature and got the state to admit homeopathy into the medical schools as part of the curriculum. The Allopaths refused to have anything to do with them. The AMA fought back hard - an extremely reactionary response. Ironically, the first editor of JAMA, Sammons, was a homeopath. He really upgraded the scientific status of the journal. The second editor, of course, was Morris Fishbein. He was just phenomenal! He was very unique, and a great storyteller. But he was not an accurate historian; you can't really take his historical writings seriously. And he was extremely reactionary politically. He was against any government involvement in organized medicine until government put a floor under doctor's fees.

After World War II, the AMA had a public relations crisis over anything to do with "socialized medicine". So they hired Whitaker and Baxter to deluge doctors and the public with propaganda, pamphlets and brochures.

In 1948, the AMA fired Fishbein as JAMA editor. He was subsequently offered six different jobs, and took them all, editorial and academic appointments. He had brought JAMA up to a high level in terms of quality. But after that, the journal went downhill for ten years with a series of editors. It wasn't until 1959 that things got better - the journal got some better editors. Now the journal is very good, under George Lundberg. It's very conscious of scientific developments and issues.

AUTHORS: How would you assess the current state of organized medicine, and the AMA?

KING: Well, for a long time the AMA was adamantly opposed to salaried physicians. I took a salaried position after the war, and I was told that it was unethical to do so. The Annual Meeting became a casualty of specialization and commercialization - it degenerated into a show for advertisers. The House of Delegates had its own policy meetings.

Now the AMA may be beginning to see the light. Its membership has been dropping, and its monopoly has been broken. So the Association is loosening up politically. It's now courting students and physicians for membership, and is considering publication of JAMA in eighteen languages.

AUTHORS: So, looking into your crystal ball, what do you think is going to happen in the future?

KING: Medicine is a victim of its own success. Doctors, of course, are paid very well. Technology is developing faster than our ability to keep up. We don't have equal access to this technology. Everyone needs constant reeducation and retraining. And doctors need so many ancillary personnel now. So the costs are simply fantastic. They can't keep increasing at this rate. On the other hand, the research and technological development continues. The crunch will come, and as a physicians' organization, the AMA will be stuck in the middle of it.

AUTHORS: How will the United States respond to this crisis?

KING: Well, Henry Adams once pointed out that in the Middle Ages, cathedral building led to objects of great beauty, but the costs nearly bankrupted many European societies. This may happen in medicine. The extreme applications of technology simply don't pay off. We have certainly reached the point of diminishing marginal utility. If we cut research budgets by 75%, the world might actually be a better place. Much of the research is garbage, anyway. It has little to do with improved patient care.

One definition of evil is "that which is self-destructive". Eventually, evil will destroy itself. We've gotten benefits, but the costs are catching up with us. Just like with Reaganomics. President Reagan may have been popular, but his presidency was one of the greatest disasters ever to befall this country.

The U.S. response will ultimately come from public awareness, particularly of the economics. So eventually the public will not support as much health care spending. We may not need as many doctors and researchers as before. But before then, the financial bottom may drop out. After all, there's nothing wrong with medicine that a good depression won't cure!

In any event, something like this will happen. This is my crystal ball, cataracts and all.

The AMA will fight a rearguard action against all of this. Now, to the Association, it's acceptable to work for a salary, and for a corporation. The patient / doctor relationship in HMOs may not be the greatest, but the public at large will either accept "second class" medical care or go without. I'm afraid that the standard of medical care may drop dreadfully. It will certainly depend on income.

AUTHORS: Any final observations about the AMA and organized medicine? The old saying is that "there will always be an England". Will there always be an AMA?

KING: Anything clear and straightforward must be wrong. Nothing, including the future, is clear. And the more you think about it, the more complex it gets. Our standards and ethics are changing in health care. Now, what is ethical is that which is good for the patient. Modern ethics really injects the doctor into the whole social realm of things. Medical ethics, as a distinct set of principles, have disappeared. So the physician, of the future will be quite different from what the AMA saw in the Nineteenth Century, or what we see now.

Yes, there will always be an AMA. But its influence, and its appearance, will probably change beyond our recognition in a relatively short period of time.

AUTHOR INDEX
By entry number.

About the Authors

Dr. James A. Johnson is Chairman and Professor in the Department of Health Services Administration and Policy and Associate Professor of Family Medicine at the Medical University of South Carolina in Charleston, S.C. He is a widely published author in the fields of behavioral and social sciences. Dr. Johnson also serves on numerous editorial boards and provides consultation to hospitals, government, and health service organizations throughout the United States.

Dr. Walter Jones is an Associate Professor in the Department of Health Services Administration and Policy at the Medical University of South Carolina. He has published extensively in the area of health policy analyisis, health politics and program evaluation. His papers have been presented at national and international conferences on public health, health administration and health services research.